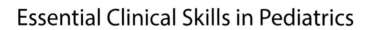

Essential Clinical Skills in Pediatrics

Anwar Qais Saadoon

Essential Clinical Skills in Pediatrics

A Practical Guide to History Taking and Clinical Examination

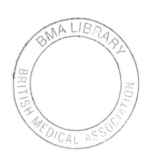

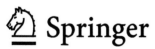

Springer

Anwar Qais Saadoon
Al-Sadr Teaching Hospital
Basra
Iraq

ISBN 978-3-319-92425-0   ISBN 978-3-319-92426-7   (eBook)
https://doi.org/10.1007/978-3-319-92426-7

Library of Congress Control Number: 2018947572

This Springer imprint is published by Springer Nature, under the registered company Springer International Publishing AG
The registered company address is: Gewerbestrasse 11, 6330 Cham, Switzerland

- *To the Iraqi people who fought terrorism, sacrificing their lives for freedom and peace. Without their sublime sacrifices, I could not have written these words for the world.*
- *To the striver Iraqi doctors who are doing their best, working day and night to treat and save the lives of millions of people, not only in Iraq but across the globe as well.*
- *To the world's best family:*
  - *My father, who taught me how to leave my imprint wherever I go.*
  - *My mother, my constant source of love and kindness. Without her warm-heartedness, I would not have been able to pass through the journey of life.*
  - *My sisters and brothers, especially Ayman, my teacher and mentor.*
- *To my dear relatives, in particular, my uncles Ali Saadoon and the great teacher Muhammad Abdallah. I will never forget their support.*
- *To all my friends, especially my soulmates, Marwan Abdulrahman and Samer Jawad.*
- *To the respectable teachers and wonderful students at Basra Medical College. I am proud to be a part of them.*
- *To those people who still live in my heart and will stay there forever.*

Foreword

Any book that is written should solve a problem. And if the book solves that problem it is worthy of publication and purchase. Such is the case of *Essential Clinical Skills in Pediatrics* by Dr. Anwar Qais. As a young medical student, Dr. Qais found that he needed a reference that would assist him in history taking and physical exam skills. That was the problem—no such reference existed. In subsequent years, and with additional training in pediatrics, he prepared a volume that solved that problem. He has done so in a fashion that is both useful and elegant.

The book, although brief, covers all the important issues in pediatrics. There are two parts: one on history-taking skills, with specific direction based on symptoms being assessed. The 31 symptoms chapters include all the pertinent topics of child healthcare, both acute and chronic complaints. The second part deals with the physical exam of the child at all stages of development. Throughout the book, there are many charts, graphs, and special lists pointing out clinical tips and key points. This makes the book very readable and user-friendly. I particularly like the fact that Dr. Qais has included pertinent points of family history and social history, which are often issues of critical importance. I also appreciated the clear instructions about setting the stage for an interview and tips on interpersonal connection with the patient and family.

This book is well written and very helpful. Instead of delivering information around a topic, it tells the reader what to do, what to ask, and what to examine. The reference section is complete and informative and serves as a starting point for more in-depth reading on particular diseases and conditions.

Indeed, Dr. Qais saw a problem and has solved it with the production of this book. I recommend his learning guide for students, residents, and practitioners of pediatrics.

Stephen Ludwig
Professor of Pediatrics
Children's Hospital of Philadelphia
Perelman School of Medicine
University of Pennsylvania
Philadelphia, PA
USA

Foreword

Anwar Qais Saadoon should be congratulated on the publication of his textbook, *Essential Clinical Skills in Pediatrics: A Practical Guide to History Taking and Clinical Examination.* The content and style are of high quality and make the information very accessible to a student or clinician who wishes to learn both the art and the science of good history taking and clinical examination.

Eliciting an accurate and complete history and the performance of a thorough and reliable clinical examination remain the foundation on which both the diagnosis and the assessment of a patient's progress are built. It is easy to forget this in these days when investigations are so readily accessible, but clinical skills will always be fundamental to medical decision making. So many times, I have seen a diagnostic problem solved by a consultation with an experienced doctor, and it is very common to see this come about when the consulted doctor returns to the basics, takes a good history, and performs a good examination.

History and examination in pediatrics pose particular challenges to the clinician's skills when the patient often cannot tell their own story, and when the examination may be influenced by the degree of cooperation. The book has very practical tips to assist with this.

This book would be very suitable for both undergraduate and postgraduate students learning pediatrics.

The key points are well emphasized. I enjoyed the introductory tips on how to prepare for the consultation.

The writing style, similar to a student's lecture notes, and the liberal use of illustrations make the content live up to the title—it is indeed both essential and practical.

Mike South
Professor of Pediatrics
University of Melbourne
Royal Children's Hospital
Murdoch Children's Research Institute
Melbourne, VIC
Australia

Foreword

"To study the phenomenon of disease without books is to sail an uncharted sea, while to study books without patients is not to go to sea at all."

—Sir William Osler

In the majority of cases, clinical diagnosis can be made on the basis of a detailed history supplemented by careful physical examination of the patient. This is the clinical method, and mastery of the clinical method is the key to the art of medicine. When the patient is a child, this is more challenging, as patients can vary from a preterm newborn to a fully grown adolescent, and medical conditions vary greatly at different ages. Moreover, in the younger child, the doctor may be faced with unwillingness of the patient to be examined and yet have the requisite skills to acquire the necessary clinical information.

Dr. Anwar Qais has produced here a very useful book, aptly entitled *Essential Clinical Skills in Pediatrics: A Practical Guide to History Taking and Clinical Examination*, as this describes exactly what the book aims to do: namely, to provide in an accessible way a concise summary of clinical pediatrics based on the practical application of the clinical method.

The first part deals with history-taking skills and symptomatology in over thirty common conditions in general pediatrics. A detailed account of the specific history to be explored in each condition is followed by key points outlining essential facts underlying these specific points in the history.

The second part deals with the physical examination of both the newborn and the older child.

The text is very readable, being presented in a lecture-note format with highlighting of important facts and supplemented with marginal notes, clinical tips, boxes, and tables where appropriate. The whole text is extremely well referenced, with over 190 references provided.

This small volume will be of great value both to undergraduate medical students and to postgraduate pediatric trainees working for their higher professional qualifications.

Peter B. Sullivan
Associate Professor of Pediatrics, Medical Sciences Division
University of Oxford, Oxford University Hospital NHS Trust
Oxford, UK

Foreword

There is no monopoly on wisdom with regard to what makes a good book. What works for one learner will not work for another, and so additions to the world literature are incredibly welcome. This new book tackles old topics with enthusiasm. At its heart, it aims to provide guidance on how to take a good history and examination. This is no small undertaking. When we asked to summarize the required undergraduate teaching for UK medical schools, we were able to condense the curriculum into the single statement: "Be able to take a history and examination, and provide basic life support for a child and/or young person." This book tackles the former in considerable detail. It differs from other books by offering detailed referencing for the interested reader, covering each system in depth.

It is with some chagrin that I have, over the years, reflected upon the lack of examination skills that I picked up in medical school. It was not until I studied for the MRCP (UK) clinical examination that I developed a "polished routine" and as I point out to students, "the sooner you learn a proper technique, the sooner you will start to gain experience." I would, therefore, advise readers to practice, practice, practice.

This book will help you to start; it acts as a beginning. Every journey requires a beginning, and this seems like a solid place to start. Only experience and repeated exposure to examination in all ages will result in mastery of physical examination. Be courageous; take careful histories and complete thorough examinations on every child you see. Commit to a diagnosis before seeking senior review and in a few years reflect on your own journey.

Will Carroll
Honorary Reader in Child Health
Chair of MRCPCH Theory Examinations, Keele University
Stoke-on-Trent, UK

Preface

"The best of people are those who are most beneficial to people."
—The Prophet Muhammad (PBUHHF)

During my study of pediatrics in the fifth year of medical college, I encountered a problem: There was no single, reliable, and concise reference pertaining to easily and comprehensively taking the history and conducting a physical examination of a newborn or older child. Such a resource would be useful in carrying out the objective structured clinical examination (OSCE). The lack of a single resource forced me to use multiple books for adequate knowledge regarding history taking and physical examination, and I had to use additional references for OSCEs. Searching multiple resources was very difficult and time-consuming. In the midst of this challenge, the idea for this book arose.

I have written this book to help others overcome the problems I had encountered. I have tried my best to make it as simple as possible. Moreover, I have striven to make this book comprehensive, informative, practical, and clinically oriented, justifying its title, *Essential Clinical Skills in Pediatrics: A Practical Guide to History Taking and Clinical Examination.*

The book is divided into two main parts, and their order has been revised to provide an intuitive structure:

- Part I discusses history-taking skills and the evaluation of the common pediatric symptoms; it contains more than 30 "History Stations," with key points, case scenarios, and many tables.
- Part II gives a close look at the clinical examination of the newborn and older child.

This book is addressed to undergraduate medical students preparing for clinical exams. It will also be helpful for a wide audience of postgraduate pediatric trainees working toward higher professional qualifications. Here is hoping that this book fulfills its aim of providing an essential and concise summary of clinical pediatric practice, not only in Iraq but in the rest of the world as well.

Basra, Iraq   Anwar Qais Saadoon

Content Reviewers

Dharmapuri Vidyasagar, MD, MSc, FAAP, FCCM, PhD (Hon)
Professor Emeritus Pediatrics
Division of Neonatology
Department of Pediatrics
College of Medicine
University of Illinois, Chicago, USA

Andrew Bush, MD, FRCP, FRCPCH, FERS
Professor of Pediatrics and Head of Section (Pediatrics), Imperial College
Professor of Pediatric Respirology, National Heart and Lung Institute
Consultant Pediatric Chest Physician, Royal Brompton & Harefield NHS Foundation
Trust, London, UK

Suraj Gupte, MD, FIAP, FSAMS (Sweden), FRSTMH (London)
Professor and Head, Postgraduate Department of Pediatrics Mamata Medical
College/Mamata General and Superspeciality Hospitals, Khammam, Telangana,
India
E-mail: drsurajgupte@gmail.com

Sergio Bernasconi, MD
Professor and Chairman, Department of Pediatrics
University of Parma, Italy

Rolando Cimaz, MD
Associate Professor of Pediatrics
University of Florence, Italy
Head of the Pediatric Rheumatology
Unit at Meyer Children's Hospital, Florence, Italy

Jamie E. Flerlage, MD, MS
Assistant Member
Department of Pediatric Oncology
St. Jude Children's Research Hospital, Memphis, TN, USA

Ming Lim, MD, PhD
Reader and Consultant Pediatric Neurologist
Division of Pediatric Neuroscience
Children's Neurosciences Center (Newcomen Center)
Evelina London Children's Hospital, King's Health Partners Academic Health Science Center, London, UK
King's College London, UK

Acknowledgements

When our emotions flow, sometimes, words are not enough to express our appreciation and gratitude. This is a fitting occasion for me to thank my mentor, Professor Khalil I. Al-Hamdi, Head of the Department of Medicine at Basra Medical College and Head of the Division of Dermatology at Al-Sadr Teaching Hospital, for his untiring support. I feel honored and privileged to have worked under his able guidance. I also wish to acknowledge the constant inspiration I have received from my teachers at Basra Medical College, who have been instrumental in not only providing my education in medical science but also in teaching me how to be an effective person in the community. I am especially indebted to Professor Thamer A. Hamdan, President of Basra University, and to Professor Ahmed M. Al-Abbasi, Dean of Basra Medical College; I also wish to give special thanks to Professor Sarkis K. Strak, who taught me the basics of the clinical method and Assistant Professor Samer A. Dhahir, who taught me how to inspect skin lesions, analyze my findings, and accurately diagnose the patient's condition.

Further, my sincere appreciation extends to the faculty of the Department of Pediatrics at Basra Medical College, and in particular, the Head of the Department, Professor Sawsan I. Habeeb, who encouraged me to put this book together; Professor Mea'ad K. Hassan; Professor Jenan G. Hassan; Assistant Professor Aida A. Manther; Dr. Baha' Al-Ethan; Dr. Assim K. Assim; Dr. Hussein J. Mohammed; Dr. Miami K. Yousif; Dr. Duha S. Jumaa; Dr. Jawad K. Atiya; Dr. Abbas A. Khazaal; Dr. Hanan R. Abood; Dr. Asa'ad I. Ashour; and Dr. Aliaa M. Radhi. I am thankful to all those great teachers who taught me the basics of pediatrics.

I would also like to state my gratitude for Professor Stephen Ludwig, Professor Mike South, Professor Peter Sullivan, Professor Hamish Wallace, Professor F. Bruder Stapleton, Professor Jeremy Friedman, and Dr. Will Carroll for their kind forewords or recommendations.

In addition, I would like to express my sincere and heartfelt thanks to all doctors at Dermatology Division and Plastic Surgery Division at Al-Sadr Teaching Hospital for their kind support.

My appreciation also extends to the brilliant copyeditor, Dr. Albert M. Liberatore; without his help and support, I could not take this book forward.

I also need to thank Dr. Samer S. Hoz and Mr. Thomas Charles, who gave me stimulating suggestions and support while I was putting this book together. Lastly, I offer my special thanks to the talented Iraqi illustrators Mohammad I. Nasser, Hussam A. Zachi, and Omar Riad for their wonderful figure sketches.

About the Book

- *Essential Clinical Skills in Pediatrics* is a concise learning guide dedicated to the full scope of pediatric history taking and clinical examination for use in OSCEs.
- Instead of delivering information about a topic, this book guides the student or clinician simply and methodically regarding what to ask when taking a history and how to perform a comprehensive physical examination.
- *ECS in Pediatrics* offers more than 30 "History Stations" covering the most common pediatric cases, as well as 10 "Examination Stations" covering examinations of the different body systems.
- The lecture-note style and the use of key points, clinical tips, notes, tables, figures, charts, and boxes listing the most important features render the book reader-friendly.
- The quick-read bulleted text and short sentences facilitate the easy-to-read format.
- *ECS in Pediatrics* contains many illustrations showing the correct way to perform clinical examinations.

About the Author

Dr. Anwar Qais Saadoon is a Resident Physician at Al-Sadr Teaching Hospital in Basra, Iraq. Graduating with distinction from the University of Basra College of Medicine in 2013, he has been a member of the Iraqi Medical Association since 2015. Dr. Qais has published several medical articles, which have been cited by numerous national and international newspapers, websites, and satellite channels. In 2015, he served as a manager of Al-Mudaina District Primary Health Care Center.

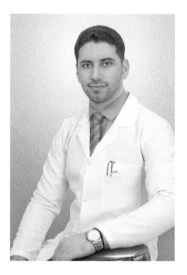

Dr. Qais has attended numerous conferences on pediatrics and conducted academic presentations in the field of pediatrics. Currently, he is pursuing a number of academic research projects and working on two books. In his free time, he enjoys reading, writing, spending time with his family in Basra, and sitting on the banks of the Euphrates, in conversation with his friends.

Contents

Part I

History-Taking Skills and Symptomatology

Basics of History Taking

1

Asking questions is the ABC of diagnosis. Only the inquiring mind solves problems.

—*Edward Hodnett*

Contents

1.1 Introduction

1. A child is sick. The parents are worried. And time is of the essence. Few moments draw upon the full scope of a doctor's knowledge and skill as when an unwell child presents with an as-yet-undiagnosed condition and needs your help. Before you can treat the condition, of course, you must diagnose what it is—and doing that will require you to take a history, carry out a relevant physical examination, and conduct investigations to confirm what the history and examination suggest. For the pediatrician, all of these are made significantly more challenging by the fact that your patient may not be capable of contributing to your diagnosis the way an adult would. Asking just the right questions and looking for all the right signs are crucial. And helping you to do that is the purpose of this book.

© Springer International Publishing AG, part of Springer Nature 2018
A. Qais Saadoon, *Essential Clinical Skills in Pediatrics*,
https://doi.org/10.1007/978-3-319-92426-7_1

3

2. Before the start of the interview, be sure to read all referral letters and past information.
3. If the child is not old enough, the best person (informant) to give the history is the child's mother or someone else closely involved in the child's care. If the child is old enough, however, you may direct questions to him or her.

> *A smart mother makes often a better diagnosis than a poor doctor.*
> —*August Bier*

4. As much as possible, take the history while sitting in a calm, "child-friendly" room.
5. Have toys accessible for children of different ages, as this will facilitate your task.
6. Be holistic in your approach to the informant and the child. Aggressiveness and a rude attitude invariably backfire, causing bottlenecks in your interview and clinical workup.
7. Introduce yourself in a friendly manner and listen carefully to the informant's or child's report. You can then ask direct questions to fill in the gaps and refine the details.
8. Talking to the child must be done in a gentle, age-appropriate manner (see Fig. 1.1) [1].
9. Call the child by his or her given name to establish a rapport. Ask if he or she has a nickname and whether the child prefers to be called by that name.
10. During the interview, observe the child's play, appearance, behavior, and gait. Such factors may help you to make a reasonable diagnosis and offer the correct management [2].
11. Maintain good eye contact with both the child and the informant. Always be friendly and maintain a respectful manner and pleasant expression.
12. Give the child and informant your full attention, listen carefully to what they say, avoid having physical barriers between you and them, and try to make them feel at ease and comfortable.
13. It is helpful to use the same structured approach every time you take a history. Such an approach ensures that important points are not missed. This increases your efficiency too [3].
14. The following structural approach is appropriate:
    - Identity (patient demographics)
    - Chief complaint(s) (presenting complaint)
    - History of present illness (history of presenting complaint)
    - Past history:
      - Birth history
        Prenatal
        Natal
        Postnatal and neonatal
      - Past medical and surgical history

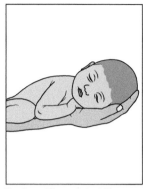

Newborn: First month of life
(first 28 days of life)

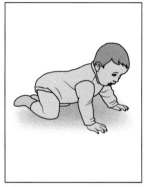

Infant: 1 to 12 months

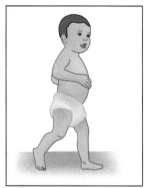

Toddler: 1 to 3 years

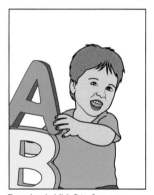

Preschool child: 3 to 6 years

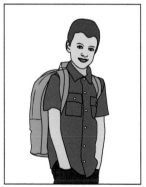

Schoolchild: 6 to 12 years
(some consider it from 5 to 18 years)

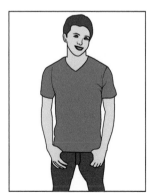

Adolescent: 12 to 18 years
(some consider adolescence
to be the period from 10 to
18 years or from 12 to 20 years)

Child: Birth to 18 years (some consider a child <15 years)

Fig. 1.1   The different ages of children

- Medication history
- Developmental history
- Immunization history
- Feeding/dietary history
- Family history
- Social history
- Review of systems

15. At the end of the interview, ask the informant whether he or she has any additional information to provide. Then thank the child and his or her family and explain the next steps.

Clinical Tips 1.1

To have effective conversations, follow these tips:
- Your words should be clear and audible.
- Start with open-ended style questions.
- Do not interrupt the informant.
- Use silence to encourage the informant to explain things.
- Try to be relaxed and unhurried.
- Do not use medical jargon during interaction with the family.
- You may need to clarify and summarize what you understand; it is better to do this more than once [4].

1.2   Identity (Patient Demographics)

A patient's identity should include the following:

1. Child's name
2. Child's age in years (with months and days) and date of birth
3. Sex of the child
4. Address and birthplace
5. Nationality, ethnicity/race
6. Name and relationship of the informant (source of information)
7. Date and time of the interview or admission
8. Source of referral

Key Points 1.1

- Knowing the child's name is important for both identification and establishment of rapport.
- Write down the child's age, because each age group has different problems and developmental achievements; consequently, the approach to a child depends on his or her age.

- Knowing the child's sex is very important because some diseases are more common or occur only in a particular sex, such as hemophilia and Duchenne muscular dystrophy (DMD), which occur almost exclusively in males.
- The child's address and birthplace are of import in the history because certain diseases are common in some areas more than in others; for example, sickle-cell disease has a high prevalence rate in sub-Saharan Africa [5].
- The question of nationality, ethnicity, and race of the child may be important because some diseases occur more in people of certain nationalities, ethnicities, or races (e.g., Kawasaki disease is more common in Japanese children and acquired lactase deficiency is more common in African-Americans and Asians.) [6]

1.3   Chief Complaint(s) (Presenting Complaint)

- The chief complaint may be a symptom, a sign, or an abnormal laboratory test result (or a combination of these items) that has caused the child or the parents to seek medical help.
- Always start with open questions, such as: "What is the main problem?" "Tell me why you are here?" "How is he/she?" "Why are you worried?" "How can I help?" These encourage the patient and the informant to open up and talk (see Box 1.1) [7].
- Clarify what they mean by any term they use, and always record the patient's (or informant's) own words.
- Note the duration of each complaint, recording the complaints in chronological order.

Box 1.1: The Three Main Styles of Questions [2, 8]

1. Open, permissive questions, such as "Tell me more about the pain," encourage the patient to talk. It is very useful to start with such questions when you are trying to find out what is going on.
2. Direct questions such as "When did the pain start?" look for a specific piece of information.
3. Leading questions such as "That is what worried you, isn't it?" may be deceptive and lead the patient to answer in an unacceptable way. No doubt, all these types of questions have their place in history taking.

If you don't ask the right questions, you don't get the right answers.
A question asked in the right way often points to its own answer.
— Edward Hodnett

1.4   History of Present Illness (History of Presenting Complaint)

Once you have identified the chief complaint, you need to find out the following:

- Type of onset (sudden or gradual)
- Duration and timing of the chief complaint
- Predisposing factors
- Site and radiation (for pain)
- Characteristics of the complaint (amount, consistency, and other features, according to the symptom; if pain, ask about its character, e.g., dull, sharp, throbbing, etc.)
- Severity of the symptom
- Frequency of attacks (if there are recurrent attacks)
- Progression of the condition (better, getting worse with time, or the same)
- Aggravating and relieving factors
- Associated symptoms
- Predicted complications
- Pertinent negative data
- Investigations that have already been done and treatments already tried
- Current state of the child (eating, drinking, passing urine or stool, sleeping, and activity)

1.5   Past History

1.5.1   Birth History

When taking the birth history, you should inquire about the factors that may affect the health of the child before, during, and after delivery. In general, you should ask about the details of birth history in all children aged less than 2 years or when these details are relevant to the child's current problem. Birth history includes the following:

Prenatal History
1. What is the mother's age? Was this pregnancy planned or not?
2. What is the number of previous pregnancies? What were the outcomes?
3. How was the mother's diet during pregnancy? Was she a smoker or an alcoholic?
4. Were there any problems or illnesses during the pregnancy? If so, in which trimester?
5. Was the mother exposed to radiation? If so, in which trimester?
6. Did she take any medication during pregnancy? If so, which medications? In which trimester?
7. When did she start antenatal care? If it was delayed, why?
8. Did she receive a tetanus vaccine?

9. How long was the pregnancy (term, preterm, post-term)?
10. Are there preexisting medical or psychiatric conditions? If so, what are they?
11. Is there any blood group incompatibility between the parents? (Rh incompatibility may cause erythroblastosis fetalis.)

Key Points 1.2

- Maternal problems or complications during pregnancy can be as follows:
  - **Infection**: HIV, rubella, syphilis, tuberculosis, hepatitis B, toxoplasmosis, etc.
  - **Illnesses**: Anemia, gestational diabetes, preeclampsia, heart diseases, etc.
  - **Abnormal vaginal bleeding**
  - **Trauma**
- Examples of toxins and teratogens: Alcohol, phenytoin, warfarin, tetracycline, narcotics, etc.
- Maternal smoking is associated with low birth weight and increased risk of obesity and diabetes in the offspring [9].

Natal History
1. How did the labor start: spontaneous or induced? If induced, why?
2. Where was the place of delivery: at home or in a hospital?
3. Who conducted the delivery: a doctor, a qualified midwife, or a nonqualified person?
4. What was the mode of delivery: vaginal or cesarean? If it was vaginal, was there any intervention needed during labor (e.g., instrumental delivery)? If it was cesarean, why?
5. What was the presentation of the fetus (e.g., breach, vertex, or face)?
6. What was the duration of the labor?
7. Were there complications during labor (such as bleeding or failure to progress)?
8. Was there maternal fever or premature rupture of membranes?
9. Did the baby have any cyanosis, asphyxia, birth trauma, or meconium aspiration?
10. When did the baby cry?

Postnatal and Neonatal History
1. What is the birth date of the child?
2. What are the birth weight and gestational age?
3. Does the informant know the initial Apgar scores? If so, what were they?
4. Were any resuscitation measures required? If so, what measures?
5. What was the method of umbilical cord cutting (if home delivery)? Who cut it, and when? Was there purulence when it was cut?
6. When was feeding initiated? How did the baby feed? Any suckling/latching difficulty?
7. Did the child receive vitamin K prophylaxis?

8. When was the first meconium passed? When was the first urine passed?
9. How was the newborn's hospital stay? Was there any problem during the hospital stay?
10. Where did he or she stay (nursery or neonatal care unit)? When was he or she discharged from the hospital? What was the age at discharge?
11. What was the infant's course in the first few weeks after discharge?
12. Were any cyanosis, jaundice, seizures, respiratory distress, infection, congenital anomalies, or birth injuries observed during the neonatal period?

Key Points 1.3

- Non-passage of meconium may imply intestinal obstruction.
- Delayed meconium passage (>24) hours may suggest cystic fibrosis.
- Absence of urine voiding in the first 2 days (48 h) of life may suggest renal agenesis or a urinary system obstruction [3].

1.5.2   Past Medical and Surgical History

In this portion of the history, you should ask the following questions:

1. How was the child's previous health? When was he or she last active and well?
2. Did the child experience similar symptoms or attacks in the past?
3. Were there previous visits to the doctor? If so, when? For what?
4. Were there any admissions to the hospital? If so, when and for what? Ask about details.
5. From what childhood illnesses and infections has the child suffered? Make a note of duration, dates, and types of various diseases.
6. Was there any recent exposure to any infectious diseases (e.g., chicken pox, measles, pertussis, or mumps)?
7. Currently, is the child on any medication? Why? Ask the informant to list them, if possible, and ask about details (see Sect. 1.6).
8. Are there any allergies? Which are they? Ask the informant to list them.
9. Was there a history of blood or blood products transfusion? If so, ask about the reason for transfusion, the date of the transfusion, the number of units, and any reactions.
10. Were there any investigations conducted in the past? If so, why? What were the results? Ask for laboratory reports, if any.
11. Does the child have a chronic illness? If so, ask about:
    - Age at diagnosis
    - Initial presentation and initial hospitalization (date, cause, duration, progression in the hospital)
    - Frequency of hospitalization (may indicate the severity of the illness)
    - Timeframe between the attacks or hospitalizations

- If the disease is controlled by a certain drug, ask in detail about that drug (see Sect. 1.6).
- Procedures, interventions, or investigations that were done for the child, as well as the results, such as:
  - Lumbar puncture and cerebrospinal fluid (CSF) analysis
  - Bone marrow (BM) biopsy or aspiration
  - Computed tomography (CT) scan or magnetic resonance imaging (MRI)
- History of last attack or admission
- Progression of the symptoms over time (better, worse, or the same)
- Impact of the chronic illness on the child and his or her family

12. Did the child undergo any surgical operations in the past? If so, at what age? For what? What type of operation? Were there any complications? If so, what were they?
13. Did the child experience an accident or injury in the past? If so, ask about the details of that event.

Key Points 1.4

- A history of recurrent diarrhea, respiratory tract infections, and sinusitis, associated with failure to thrive in spite of good food intake, strongly suggest cystic fibrosis [10].
- Acute wheezing in a child, with similar attacks in the past, is highly suggestive of bronchial asthma [3].

1.6   Medication History

A careful medication history is vital for preventing prescription errors and detecting problems that may be induced or aggravated by a medication. In addition, it may be important in identifying changes in clinical signs that may result from a certain medication. To take an accurate medication history, find out:

1. Is the child on any medication? If so, why? What are the current medications that the child uses? For each one, take note of the following:
   - What is the drug's name? Form? Route of the administration?
   - What is the duration of treatment?
   - What are the dosages and timing of administration?
   - Are there any new dosage adjustments?
   - What is the frequency of administration?
   - Who is responsible for the drug administration?
   - Is the drug actually taken as prescribed (compliance)?
   - Are there any side effects/adverse drug reactions (ADRs)? Allergies?
   - Is there proper storage of the drug?
2. Is there a relevant recent drug (e.g., courses of steroids for asthma)?

3. Has there been a recent long-term use of antibiotics?
4. Are there any allergies to medications or food or previous significant drug side effects?
5. Are there any non-medicine or non-prescribed drugs (e.g., vitamins and herbal preparations)?
6. Ask about drugs that may be relevant to the current condition (e.g., anticoagulants may cause bleeding tendency; NSAIDs may cause gastric ulceration or upper-gastrointestinal bleeding).
7. If the child uses home nebulizers, you must note the method of mixing and administration of the medications and diluent. Ask about the devices that are used for the drug administration and inquire about the used technique (i.e., open-mouth or closed-mouth technique).

> *The young physician starts life with 20 drugs for each disease,*
> *and the old physician ends life with one drug for 20 diseases.*
> — *Sir William Osler*

Clinical Tips 1.2

- If the parents say that their child has a drug allergy, clarify exactly what they mean by the word "allergy."
- Allergies to drugs are often overreported by parents.
- A penicillin skin test is positive in only one of seven patients who report a skin rash after penicillin use [4].

1.7   Developmental History

Assessment of the child's development consists of two parts: **Developmental history** (discussed here) and **observation** of developmental progress through physical examination.

1. Start with these important questions:
   - What are the details of the present skills?
   - Are there any concerns about the child's development, vision, or hearing?
   - Has there been any regression or delay in milestones? If so, is the child's development globally delayed or only in a particular field?
   - If there is a global delay, then ask if it is progressive or nonprogressive.
   - If the delay is in an individual field, ask which developmental domain is delayed.
2. Find out the age at which major milestones were achieved for the four developmental areas (Fig. 1.2):
   - Gross motor
   - Fine motor and vision

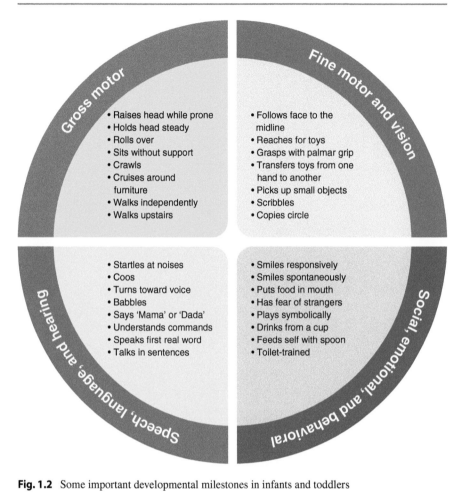

Fig. 1.2   Some important developmental milestones in infants and toddlers

- Speech, language, and hearing
- Social, emotional, and behavioral

3. Compare these milestones with those of older siblings at the same age.
4. Ask about the child's playing and interaction with children of his/her age or younger.
5. It is also important to ask about school grade and work quality in school-aged children.
6. Ask about any period of growth failure, unusual growth, or asymmetry in body growth.
7. It is very important to understand the normal developmental milestones, especially if you suspect a developmental delay or arrest. Standard developmental milestones are summarized in Tables 1.1 and 1.2.

Table 1.1 Developmental milestones in the first 10 months of life [2, 11–15]

Age	Gross motor	Fine motor and vision	Speech, language, and hearing	Social, emotional, and behavioral
Newborn	Limbs flex; symmetrical posture; head flat in prone	Hands close symmetrically; follows face and light to the midline	Alerts at bell; **startles at loud noises**; cries	Regards face
2 months	Raises head while prone; starts to lift chest	Follows object moved vertically, when supine	**Coos** (2–4 months); searches for sound with eyes	**Smiles responsively** (4–8 weeks); recognizes parent
4 months	Pulls to sit, with no head lag (3 months); **holds the head steady; rolls to supine**	Hands open (3–4 months); brings objects to mouth; **reaches for objects** palmar grasp (4–6 months)	Laughs and squeals; **turns toward voice**	**Smiles spontaneously**; excited at site of food
6 months	**Sits without support, with round back;** asymmetric tonic neck reflex fully inhibited	**Palmar grasp of objects**; reaches for toys with one-hand approach and grasp	Monosyllabic babbles (consonant sounds)	**Puts food in mouth** (6–8 months)
7 months	**Rolls over** (6.5 months); creep-crawls	**Transfers toys from one hand to another** (5.5–7 months)	Turns to soft sounds out of sight; sounds used indiscriminately; **polysyllabic babble**	Favors mother; responds to changes in emotional content of social contact; enjoys mirror
8 months	**Sits without support, with straight back; crawls** (8–9 months)	Thumb-finger grasp	Understands "no" when strongly spoken; responds to name when called (turns)	Holds own bottle; finger feeds
10 months	**Walks around furniture;** lets self down from standing, with partial control	**Mature pincer grip**	Says "Mama" or "Dada"; points to objects; follows one-step command without gesture	**Fear of strangers** (7–10 months); **waves "bye-bye"**; plays "peekaboo" (10–12 months)

Table 1.2 Developmental milestones from 1 to 6 years [2, 11–15]

Age	Gross motor	Fine motor and vision	Speech, language, and hearing	Social, emotional, and behavioral
1 year	**Rises independently; walks unsteadily, broad gait, hands apart**	**Turns pages of book; releases object on command**	**Speaks first real word;** says two to three words other than "Dada" or "Mama"	**Imitates actions; drinks from a cup with two hands;** points to indicate wants; comes when called
15 months	**Walks independently; crawls upstairs**	**Scribbles** (13–15 months); immature grip of pencil	**4–6 words; follows command without gesture**	Asks for objects by pointing
18 months	**Walks up steps**	Makes marks with a crayon (16–18 months); **builds a tower of three**	6–10 words; shows two parts of the body	**Feeds self with spoon; symbolic play (18–24 months)**
2 years	**Runs well**; jumps; kicks ball	**Builds a tower of six; draws a horizontal line**	**Uses two or more words to make simple phrases**	**Dry by day; pulls off some clothing;** verbalizes wants
2.5 years	Rides tricycle using pedals	**Builds a tower of eight or a train with four bricks**	**Names all body parts; knows full name**	Pulls up pants; washes, dries hands
3 years	Throws ball overhand; **walks upstairs** (alternating feet)	**Builds a bridge (from a model); copies circle; draws a cross (3.5 years)**	**Talks constantly in 3–4 word sentences; knows age and sex**	Parallel play; interactive play evolving; **toilet trained**
4 years	Hops on one foot	**Builds steps (after demonstration); copies square**	**Understands prepositions;** asks "how" and "why"; **tells story**	**Dresses with little assistance; shoes on correct feet;** plays out with other children
5 years	Skips (alternating feet); walks on a line; comes downstairs one at a time	**Draws a triangle;** writes own name; does up buttons	**Names 4 colors;** repeats sentence of 10 syllables; fluent speech; **knows date of birth**	**Ties shoelaces;** chooses own friends; identifies coins; **dresses without supervision**
6 years	Jumps with feet together	**Draws a diamond**	Knows address and telephone number	**Can discriminate right and left**

1.8   Immunization History

When taking the immunization history, you may need to ask the following questions:

1. Is the child up-to-date with his/her immunizations? Did he/she complete the immunizations suggested for his/her age (according to the national immunization schedule)? What immunizations have been received?
2. Were there any missed or omitted vaccines? If so, what were they? Why?
3. Were there any adverse events/effects in relation to immunization? If so, what were they? When did they occur? To which vaccines were they related?
4. Is there an allergy to any vaccine? If so, to which vaccine?
5. Did the child receive booster dose(s) of vaccine(s)? If so, what were they? What are the dates of recent boosters?
6. Did the child receive any optional vaccines? If so, what were they? When were they given? Why?

Notes 1.1

- It is very important to see any related documentation, such as immunization records from the primary healthcare provider or the parents' own shot records. This may be of benefit in the verification of compliance with the national immunization schedule.
- In certain parts of the world, you may need to ask about the BCG scar and recent tuberculosis testing results.
- In many countries, there are multiple national immunization days (NIDs) and subnational immunization days (SNIDs). These are a part of the enhanced immunization campaigns and are conducted in addition to a routine national immunization schedule.
- Many communicable diseases, especially polio and measles, are targeted by these immunization campaigns.
- Since the immunization campaigns do not substitute for routine immunizations, every child should be immunized according to the national immunization schedule, regardless of the immunization campaigns.

1.9   Feeding/Dietary History

The feeding and dietary history should establish the quantity and quality of the diet that is consumed by the child. In addition, it should determine the eating behaviors of the child and beliefs of his/her family.

1.9.1 For an Infant

Find out whether he or she is breastfed or taking formula, and then ask about the method of feeding.

1. **Breastfeeding**
   Ask the following questions:
   - What is the duration of exclusive breastfeeding?
   - Is breastfeeding on demand or scheduled?
   - What is the frequency of breastfeeding?
   - How often does the child feed at night?
   - What is the duration of each feeding?
   - What is the feeding technique that the mother uses? (see Box 1.2)
   - Does the mother use both breasts for feeding?
   - Is the feeding adequate to the child (sleeping after feeding; weight gain; passing urine)?
   - Is there excessive crying?
   - Are there any feeding difficulties (e.g., choking, regurgitation, or vomiting)?
   - Are there any worries regarding breastfeeding (e.g., anxiety regarding the adequacy of milk supply, return to work, or breast pain/discomfort due to sore nipples, mastitis, or thrush)?
   - Does the mother wash her hands before and after each feeding?
   - Did the child receive vitamins or mineral supplements?
   - Did the mother start complementary feeding? If so, what? At what age?

Box 1.2: Tips for Breastfeeding [3, 12]

- There are many feeding positions. In all of them, the mother should be comfortable and relaxed.
- The infant's face and body should be close and facing the breast.
- The infant's body should be supported straight in the same plane with the head.
- The infant's chin should touch the mother's breast, with his nose opposite to the nipple.
- The infant's mouth should be wide open, with the lower lip everted and much of the areola inside the mouth.
- Remember, the essential components of the infant's proper latching (attachment) are:
  - Wide-open mouth
  - Everted lower lip
  - Most of the areola in infant's mouth
  - Chin touching the breast

Notes 1.2

- Breastfeeding should be started as early as possible, preferably within half an hour of childbirth; it is preferred for the first 2 years of life (exclusively for the first 6 months; no water should be given, even in hot weather) [12, 16].
- On-demand feeding means feeding the infant on every occasion he/she cues that he/she is hungry.
- Initially, breastfed babies suckle for 5 min on each breast. This process may be repeated every 1–3 h. Subsequently, nursing time can be increased to 10–15 min on each breast [16, 17].
- Most newborns sleep for up to 5 h. In this period of time, they will not need to be fed [17].
- Adequacy of breastfeeding can be assessed by adequate weight gain, adequate sleeping (2–3 h) after each feeding, voiding of urine six to eight times/day, and passage of loose yellow stool at least four times per day (by 5–7 days). (Note that exclusively breastfed babies may stool only once every 3–5 days, which is still normal) [12, 16–18].
- Up to 10% (15% in preterm newborns) of birth weight may be lost in the first 5–7 days of life. This should be regained by 10 days. In general, by 4–5 months of life, weight is doubled, and by 1 year, it is tripled. Weight gain in the first 3 months of life is about 30 g/day [12, 17, 18].
- The American Academy of Pediatrics (AAP) recommends 8–12 feedings per day (or more frequently) at the breast for healthy term infants [19, 20].
- Frequent uninterrupted breastfeeding, as well as feeding at night, can increase milk production and can help prevent the problem of not having enough milk [21].
- Vitamin D supplementation (400 IU/day) is recommended by the American Academy of Pediatrics (AAP) for all breastfed infants; it should be started at birth and continued throughout the first year of life [18].

2. **Formula Feeding**
   - When did formula feeding start?
   - What type of milk is used?
   - How is it prepared? Is it diluted?
   - What is the mode of feeding (i.e., bottle-fed or Katori spoon-fed)?
   - How much milk does the child consume in each feeding (in ounces)?
   - What is the volume of the residual milk?
   - What is the frequency of feeding?
   - What is the average duration of each feeding?
   - Are there any feeding problems (e.g., allergies, diarrhea, or colic)?
   - Is there any change in bowel habits?
   - Is the feeding adequate for the child (sleeping after feeding, weight gain, passing urine)?

- How many bottles does the mother have?
- What is the method of sterilization used?
- Did the mother introduce semisolids or solids? If so, when? What are they?

Notes 1.3

- As a guiding principle, formula feeding needs to be discouraged.
- The frequency of formula feeding is variable (depending on gastric emptying time). It should be regulated by the infants themselves "on demand." Most infants will demand 6–9 feedings per day after the first week of life; they may nurse every 2–4 h. The volume of feedings may be rapidly increased from 1 to 3 ounces (about 30–90 mL) every 3–4 h by the end of the first week of life [22, 23].
- Infants should receive at least 16 ounces (480 mL) of formula per day at 1 year of age [17].
- Formulas contain 20 kcal/oz. (0.67 kcal/mL) when prepared correctly [21].
- Unmodified cow's milk and honey should be avoided in infants less than 12 months of age [24, 25].

3. *Weaning*
   - When were complementary foods first introduced? At what age? (see Box 1.3)
   - What is the nature of weaning foods? (Type of weaning foods)?
   - When were gluten-containing foods (e.g., biscuits, bread containing wheat as gluten) first introduced? At what age?
   - How were weaning foods administered (i.e., by spoon or in a bottle)?
   - What is the amount of food given to the child per day?
   - Does the child feed on demand or on a schedule? What is the frequency of food intake?
   - Does the child suck or swallow well? At what age did he/she start to manage lumpy food?
   - Did he/she have any preference?
   - Were there any known allergies to weaning food? If so, to which food?
   - Did the mother face any problems during weaning? If so, how did she deal with them?

Box 1.3: Complementary Foods

- The World Health Organization (WHO) defines complementary foods as "any food, whether manufactured or locally prepared, suitable as a complement to breast milk or to a breast-milk substitute, when either becomes insufficient to satisfy the nutritional requirements of the infant." [26]
- The suitable time for complementary foods introduction is just beyond 6 months of age [16, 27].
- New-food introduction should take place one at a time, with observation for any allergies for 2–3 days after introduction [25].

- The addition of salt and sugar to complementary foods should be avoided [27].
- Introduction of foods with high allergenicity (such as egg whites, berries, and nuts) should be avoided until 1 year of age [28].
- Introduced complementary foods should be soft, fresh homemade, affordable, easily available, and well tolerated [12, 16].

1.9.2 For Older Children

1. What was the child's food intake during the 24 h before the onset of illness?
2. How many meals and snacks per 24 h?
3. What is the current composition of the child's diet?
4. What are the favorite foods for the child?
5. Is the child forbidden to have a particular food? If so, why?
6. Did the child receive vitamin and micronutrient (e.g., fluoride) supplements? If so, record the dose.
7. Are there any problems associated with feeding (e.g., difficulty feeding, regurgitation, or vomiting)?
8. Is there any food allergy (e.g., cow milk, egg, or soybean)?
9. Are there any odd behaviors associated with eating?
10. Is the feeding adequate for the child (weight gain, sleeping, activity)?
11. Is there a history of eating nonedible things, such as clay, chalk, paper, paint, hair, etc. (pica)?

1.10 Family History

In this important part of the history, you need to find out:

1. The history of each parent: Name, age, and health.
2. The degree of consanguinity between the parents (see Box 1.4).
3. Siblings: Number, age, sex, illnesses, disabilities, and significant medical history of all siblings.
4. Birth order of the child in the family.
5. Similar problem in the family.
6. History of death among the parents or siblings; if so, ask about cause, age, and date of death.
7. Illnesses that run in the family.
8. Diseases that affect more than one member of the family.
9. Drawing out of a family tree. If there is a positive family history of genetic disorder or inborn error of metabolism (IEM), extend the family pedigree over several generations (see Fig. 1.3 and Box 1.5).

10. Chronic diseases in the family (e.g., atopy, asthma, seizures, diabetes, heart diseases, headaches, inflammatory bowel disease (IBD), deafness, etc.).

Box 1.4: Degrees of Consanguinity [3]

- **First degree**: parents, siblings (brothers and sisters), or children (sons and daughters). First-degree relatives share 50% of their genes.
- **Second degree**: uncles, aunts, nephews, nieces, grandparents, grandchildren, or half-siblings. Second-degree relatives share 25% of their genes.
- **Third degree**: first-cousins, great-grandparents, or great-grandchildren. Third-degree relatives share 12.5% of their genes.

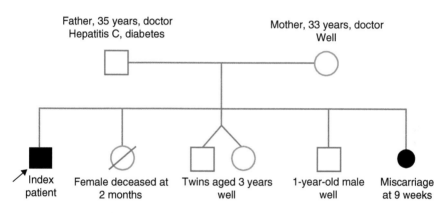

Fig. 1.3   Example of family pedigree

Box 1.5: Pedigree Symbols

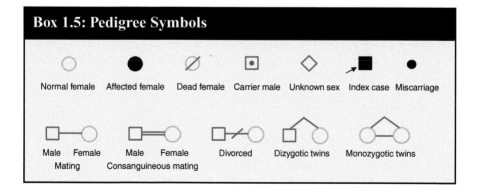

1.11   Social History

This part of the history describes the relationship of the child with his or her family, environment, and school.

1. Parents: Education level, occupation, and smoking. Do parents live together?
2. Other family members: Who lives with the child at home? Who are the main caregivers? What is the quality of the child's relationships with them?
3. What is the quality of interaction with peers (in and out of school), teachers, sibling(s), and parents?
4. Which school does the child attend? What school and play facilities are offered for the child? Has there been a similar illness in children attending the same class?
5. Who are the child's friends? What is the quality of his/her relationships with them? Are there any problems with them?
6. Does the child have any hobbies? What are they?
7. What are the child's worries or stresses?
8. Ask about housing and living conditions:
   - Where and how does the family live?
   - Do they own or rent their home?
   - How many rooms does the home have? Is it overcrowded? Ask about the number of people living in the patient's house.
   - Ask about the water and electricity supplies.
   - Ask about sanitary conditions and safety measures (running water, toilet, etc.).
9. Ask about financial support: What is the family income?
10. Ask about any history of traveling in relation to the onset of illness.
11. Inquire whether there has been contact with a patient who has the same symptoms.
12. Ask about animal relationships and pet rearing. Which kinds of pets (cat, dog, bird, etc.)?
13. In adolescents, you may need to ask about marital status, sexual activity, smoking, alcohol, and drug abuse.

Key Points 1.5

- Traveling represents an important source of infectious diseases, such as hepatitis A, typhoid fever, tuberculosis, poliomyelitis, cholera, malaria, schistosomiasis, diphtheria, and Ebola virus.
- Contact with animals can transmit many diseases (e.g., brucellosis, salmonellosis, toxoplasmosis, rabies, etc.).

1.12   Review of Systems (ROS)

The purpose of the review of systems is to be sure you have not missed anything. It is of vital importance that you orient this portion of the history to matters relevant to the child's complaint and suitable to his/her age, rather than asking about a long

Table 1.3 Review of systems [2, 3, 8, 25, 29–31]

The system	Common symptoms
General	General health, sleep disturbance, activity (decreased or increased), school absence, weight loss/gain, fever, or decreased appetite
Neurological	Headache, dizziness, vertigo, fainting, loss of consciousness, postural deformities, weakness, convulsion, anosmia, tremor, or paresthesia
Visual	Visual disturbance, ocular pain, itchy eyes, red eyes, abnormal tearing, or eye discharge
Ears, nose, and throat (ENT)	Earache, tinnitus, hearing impairment, ear discharge, recurrent sore throat, epistaxis, runny nose, sneezing, mouth breathing, or snoring
Cardiovascular	Chest pain, dyspnea, orthopnea, paroxysmal nocturnal dyspnea (PND), palpitation, fainting, fatigue, cyanosis, feeding difficulties, sweating, or edema
Respiratory	Chest pain, dyspnea, fast breathing, grunting, cyanosis, cough, sputum, hemoptysis, wheezing, stridor, or choking
Gastrointestinal	Appetite (increased or decreased), abdominal pain, abdominal mass, altered bowel motion (diarrhea or constipation), nausea, vomiting, flatulence, swallowing difficulties, jaundice, hematemesis, melena, or bleeding per rectum
Genitourinary	Frequency of urination, dysuria, hematuria, polyuria/oliguria, change in urine color, character of the urine stream, bedwetting, urethral or vaginal discharge, vaginal bleeding, age of menarche, or dysmenorrhea
Musculoskeletal	Joint pain, joint swelling, joint stiffness, joint locking, muscle weakness, muscles pain, deformity, bone pain, or disturbance of gait
Endocrine	Growth delay, neck swelling, polyphagia, excessive thirst/fluid intake, obesity, or decreased activity
Skin, hair, and nails	Rashes, itching, bruising, lumps/bumps, or nails/hair changes

list of routine but purposeless items. The most important symptoms relating to different systems are listed in Table 1.3.

References

1. Gill D, O'Brien N. Pediatric clinical examination made easy. 6th ed. Edinburgh: Elsevier; 2018.
2. Lissauer T, Macaulay C. History and examination. In: Lissauer T, Carroll W, editors. Illustrated textbook of pediatrics. 5th ed. Edinburgh: Elsevier; 2018. p. 9–26.
3. Gupte S, Smith R. Pediatric history-taking and clinical examination. In: Gupte S, editor. The short textbook of pediatrics. 12th ed. New Delhi: Jaypee Brothers Medical Publishers; 2016. p. 19–37.
4. Snadden D, Laing R, Potts S, Nicol F, Colledge N. History taking and general examination. In: Douglas G, Nicol F, Robertson C, editors. Macleod's clinical examination. 13th ed. Edinburgh: Elsevier; 2013. p. 1–63.
5. Rosse SD, Odame I, Atrash HK, Amendah DD, Piel FB, Williams TN. Sickle cell disease in Africa: a neglected cause of early childhood mortality. Am J Prev Med. 2011;41(6 Suppl 4):S398–405. https://doi.org/10.1016/j.amepre.2011.09.013.
6. Gershman G. Diarrhea. In: Berkowitz CD, editor. Berkowitz's pediatrics a primary care approach. 4th ed. Elk Grove Village, IL: American Academy of Pediatrics; 2012. p. 699–703.

7. Brugha R, Marlais M, Abrahamson E. Pocket tour pediatrics clinical examination. London: JP Medical; 2013.
8. Kulkarni ML. Clinical methods in pediatrics: history taking and symptomatology, vol. 1. New Delhi: Jaypee Brothers Medical Publishers; 2005.
9. Svoren BM, Joseph N. Diabetes mellitus. In: Kleigman RM, Stanton BF, Schor NF, St Geme III JW, Behrman RE, editors. Nelson textbook of pediatrics. 20th ed. Philadelphia: Elsevier; 2016. p. 2760–90.
10. McColley SA. Respiratory disorders. In: Green TP, Franklin WH, Tanz R, editors. Pediatrics just the facts. New York: McGraw-Hill; 2005. p. 519–38.
11. Newell SJ, Darling JC. Pediatrics lecture notes. 9th ed. Chichester: Wiley; 2014.
12. Narang M. Approach to practical pediatrics. 2nd ed. New Delhi: Jaypee Brothers Medical Publishers; 2011.
13. Feigelman S. The first year. In: Kleigman RM, Stanton BF, Schor NF, St Geme III JW, Behrman RE, editors. Nelson textbook of pediatrics. 20th ed. Philadelphia: Elsevier; 2016. p. 65–70.
14. Cvetnic WG, Pino E. USMLE step 2 CK pediatrics lecture notes. New York: Kaplan; 2013.
15. Mehra T. Pre NEET pediatrics. New Delhi: Jaypee Brothers Medical Publishers; 2013.
16. Tiwari SK, Gupte S, Gomez EM. Infant and young child feeding. In: Gupte S, editor. The short textbook of Pediatrics. 12th ed. New Delhi: Jaypee Brothers Medical Publishers; 2016. p. 1183–96.
17. Dusenbery SM, White AJ. Patient care. In: Dusenbery SM, White AJ, editors. The Washington manual of pediatrics. Philadelphia: Lippincott Williams & Wilkins; 2009. p. 1–10.
18. Buchanan AO, Marquez ML. Diet of the normal infant. In: Marcdante KJ, Kliegman RM, editors. Nelson essentials of pediatrics. 7th ed. Philadelphia: Elsevier; 2015. p. 86–9.
19. American Academy of Pediatrics. Section on breastfeeding: breastfeeding and the use of human milk. Pediatrics. 2012. http://pediatrics.aappublications.org/content/early/2012/02/22/peds.2011-3552. Accessed 5 Dec 2017.
20. Parks EP, Shaikhkhalil A, Groleau V, Wendel D, Stallings VA. Feeding healthy infants, children, and adolescents. In: Kleigman RM, Stanton BF, Schor NF, St Geme III JW, Behrman RE, editors. Nelson textbook of pediatrics. 20th ed. Philadelphia: Elsevier; 2016. p. 286–95.
21. Nigam KS. Not enough milk. In: Thora S, Goswami VP, Yewale V, Jain H, Rawat SS, Malpani P, et al., editors. Pediatrics for practitioner. New Delhi: Jaypee Brothers Medical Publishers; 2014. p. 15–20.
22. Phillips SM, Jensen C. Dietary history and recommended dietary intake in children. In: Motil KJ, Hoppin AG, editors. UpToDate. 2016. https://www.uptodate.com/contents/dietary-history-and-recommended-dietary-intake-in-children. Accessed 4 Jan 2018.
23. McCallum Z, Bines J. Nutrition. In: South M, Isaacs D, editors. Practical pediatrics. 7th ed. Edinburgh: Elsevier; 2012. p. 61–75.
24. Sidwell RU, Thomson MA. Easy pediatrics. Boca Raton: CRC Press; 2011.
25. Feinberg AN, Davidson N, Tsitsika A. Taking a history in infants, children, and adolescents. In: Greydanus DE, Feinberg AN, Patel DR, Homnick DN, editors. The pediatric diagnostic examination. New York: McGraw-Hill; 2008. p. 1–23.
26. World Health Organization. Strengthening action to improve feeding of infants and youngchildren 6–23 months of age in nutrition and child health programmes. Geneva: World Health Organization; 2008. http://www.who.int/maternal_child_adolescent/documents/9789241597890/en. Accessed 5 Dec 2017.
27. Fewtrill M. Complementary foods. In: Koletzko B, Bhatia J, Bhutta ZA, Cooper P, Makrides M, Uauy R, et al., editors. Pediatric nutrition in practice: world review of nutrition and dietetics, vol. 113. 2nd ed. Basel: Nestec Ltd; 2015. p. 109–12.
28. Dilley K, Sanguino S. Pediatric history and physical. In: Green TP, Franklin WH, Tanz R, editors. Pediatrics just the facts. New York: McGraw-Hill; 2005. p. 7–11.

29. Tasker RC, McClure RJ, Acerini CL. Oxford handbook of pediatrics. 2nd ed. Oxford: Oxford University Press; 2013.
30. Elizabeth K, Albright MD. Current clinical strategies: pediatric history and physical examination. 4th ed. California: Current Clinical Strategies Publishing; 2003.
31. Stephenson T, Wallace H, Thomson A. Clinical pediatrics for postgraduate examination. 3rd ed. Edinburgh: Elsevier Science Limited; 2002.

History Taking of Common Pediatric Cases

2

> *Listen to the patient, he is telling you the diagnosis.*
>
> —*Sir William Osler*

Contents

© Springer International Publishing AG, part of Springer Nature 2018
A. Qais Saadoon, *Essential Clinical Skills in Pediatrics*,
https://doi.org/10.1007/978-3-319-92426-7_2

2.1   Introduction

- The diagnosis of a patient's problem is mainly based on careful history taking. Hence, it is crucial to gather accurate information and data regarding the patient's presenting complaint(s) and further history.
- Since it may be difficult for pediatric patients to communicate well about their complaints, you must listen well to them with considerable patience, pay attention to what they say, and understand their responses. Thereafter, you should seek clarification and additional information from their parents or caregivers.
- This chapter will help you to apply the detailed format introduced in the first chapter to the analysis of each individual patient's complaint. It focuses on common pediatric problems, including the most pertinent topics in child healthcare, with regard to both acute and chronic complaints, offering more than 30 history stations, each station followed by key points underpinning important points in the history.
- The history stations contain comprehensive lists of questions covering the most common or important possibilities. Therefore, your history must be tailored accordingly. You may need to exercise initiative in picking appropriate questions as indicated by the patient's age and sex and, when appropriate, the suspected diagnosis.
- Additionally, this chapter will provide you with detailed tables containing the main short case scenarios and differential diagnoses for the most important childhood problems.

2.2   Dyspnea

- **Dyspnea (shortness of breath)** can be defined as a subjective uncomfortable feeling of having difficult and labored respiration, usually manifested as increased work of breathing [1].
- It can be caused by a variety of pulmonary, cardiac, or systemic disorders.

History Station 2.1: Dyspnea

- **Identity:** Age
- **Chief complaint:** Shortness of breath
- **History of present illness:**
  1. Onset: Sudden (e.g., inhaled foreign body, lung collapse), gradual (e.g., asthma, diabetic ketoacidosis)
  2. Duration
  3. Timing of dyspnea: Does the child ever awake with breathlessness?
  4. What was the child doing at the time of onset (if acute)?
  5. Frequency of attacks of dyspnea

Continued on the next page

6. Severity: Does shortness of breath restrict the child's daily activities? If so, to what degree (e.g., dyspnea only during activity, interferes with usual activities, at rest, interferes with speech, the child is too dyspneic to speak)?
7. Aggravating or relieving factors: Exercise, perfume, dust, certain positions, bronchodilators
8. Associated symptoms: Cough (duration in days), sputum and hemoptysis, fever, chest pain, sore throat, runny nose (may suggest infectious cause), abnormal breath sound, cyanosis, etc.

- **Past history:**
  A—Birth history: Maternal age, gestational diabetes, maternal chorioamnionitis, mode of delivery (if it was cesarean section (CS), ask whether it was elective or emergency CS), any intervention needed during labor, prolonged labor, meconium-stained amniotic fluid (MSAF), a history of birth asphyxia, gestational age, birth weight, twinning, prenatal ultrasonographic findings (e.g., structural lung abnormalities or oligohydramnios)
  B—Past medical and surgical history: Asthma, recurrent wheeze, diabetes, congenital heart disease, heart failure, cardiomyopathy or other cardiac problem, hypertension, eczema, allergy, history of blood transfusion, history of choking, a similar attack in the past, etc. If the condition is recurrent, ask about the age of onset of the first attack, triggers, frequency, severity of previous episodes, previous hospitalization or ICU admissions, and previous tests (X-rays, echocardiograms, ECGs, pulmonary function testing, etc.)
- **Medication history:** Beta-blockers, response to bronchodilators, corticosteroids, digoxin, furosemide, salicylate overdose, and allergies
- **Immunization history:** Bacillus Calmette–Guérin (BCG); diphtheria, pertussis, and tetanus (DPT); measles/measles, mumps, and rubella (MMR); oral polio vaccine (OPV)/inactivated polio vaccine (IPV); hepatitis B and A; *Haemophilus influenzae* type B (Hib); varicella, pneumococcal, rotavirus vaccines
- **Feeding/dietary history:** Feeding difficulty, fast breathing or diaphoresis with feedings, prolonged feeding time, and reduced volume of feeding
- **Family history:** Family history of asthma, allergies, atopic dermatitis, congenital heart disease
- **Social history**: Traveling, overcrowded house, anyone at home who has respiratory symptoms (suggests infectious cause), pollution/use of wood or coal for cooking at home, smoking (active or passive), drug addiction (heroin and other opioids)
- **Review of systems:** Itching, rash, pallor, night sweats, poor weight gain, diarrhea, vomiting, seizures, limb weakness, headache, etc.

Key Points 2.1

- Knowing the child's age is important because causes of dyspnea may vary with age.
- Dyspnea with chest pain may suggest **pneumothorax, rib fractures from trauma**, or **pleurisy**.
- Fever suggests **an infectious etiology** (pneumonia, pleural effusion, or bronchitis).
- Sudden onset of dyspnea may suggest **an inhaled foreign body** or **lung collapse**.
- Dyspnea of **asthma** or **diabetic ketoacidosis** usually develops over several hours.
- **Orthopnea** is dyspnea that worsens on lying flat. It is often caused by **left-ventricular failure, obstructive airway disease**, or **muscle weakness**.
- **Platypnea** is shortness of breath that occurs in the upright position and is alleviated by lying in a supine position. In general, it is the result of **intracardiac, vascular**, or **parenchymal lung shunts**.
- Heroin can cause **bronchospasm** that can be relieved by bronchodilators. Furthermore, it can infrequently precipitate **non-cardiogenic pulmonary edema (acute respiratory distress syndrome)** [2].

2.3　Cyanosis

- **Cyanosis** is a bluish discoloration of the skin, mucous membranes, or nailbeds.
- It is usually caused by an increment in the concentration of unsaturated hemoglobin.
- Cyanosis may be central or peripheral in origin.
- Any child with cyanosis requires careful assessment to exclude congenital or acquired respiratory or cardiac diseases.
- Respiratory disorders are the most common cause of life-threatening cyanosis in children [3].

History Station 2.2: Cyanosis

- **Identity:** Age (newborn or older child; see below)
- **Chief complaint:** Cyanosis, a bluish discoloration of the skin, lips, mucous membranes, or nailbeds
- **History of present illness:**
  1. Onset of cyanosis: Sudden or gradual
  2. Duration
  3. Timing of cyanosis
  4. Location: What parts of the body are involved?
  5. Frequency of cyanotic episode

Continued on the next page

6. Continuous or intermittent
7. Associated symptoms: Dyspnea, cough, wheezing, stridor, fever, excessive crying
8. Precipitating, aggravating, and relieving factors—exercise, feeding, crying, special positions, etc.
9. Chest trauma

- **Past history:**
  A—Birth history: Maternal diabetes, maternal drug use during pregnancy, polyhydramnios, oligohydramnios, ruptured membrane, prolonged labor, meconium-stained amniotic fluid, a history of birth asphyxia, gestational age, birth weight
  B—Past medical and surgical history: Previous episodes of cyanosis, child's age when the first episode of cyanosis occurred, congenital heart disease, prior lung disease (e.g., asthma), neurological diseases like seizures or neuromuscular disease

- **Medication history:** Recent use of medications (e.g., amiodarone), medications that may cause methemoglobinemia (e.g., antibiotics sulphonamides, antimalarial drugs)

- **Developmental history:** Has the child's development and growth been normal?

- **Feeding/dietary history:** Feeding difficulty, fast breathing or diaphoresis with feedings, prolonged feeding time

- **Family history:** Family history of asthma, hemoglobinopathy, congenital heart disease, or birth defects

- **Social history:** Contact with anyone who has an infectious disease, drug abuse, exposure to oxidant toxins, smoke inhalation, or cold exposure

Key Points 2.2

In newborns:
- **Maternal diabetes** may be associated with **cyanotic congenital heart disease, neonatal hypoglycemia**, and **neonatal polycythemia**.
- **Polyhydramnios** is associated with **fetal airway, esophageal**, and **neurological conditions**.
- **Oligohydramnios** may be associated with **pulmonary hypoplasia** and **renal defects**.
- **Meconium staining of the amniotic fluid** is associated with **meconium aspiration syndrome** and **persistent pulmonary hypertension** [3].

In older children:

- Persistent cyanosis may be caused by **congenital heart disease, primary lung disease, pulmonary artery hypertension**, or **abnormal hemoglobin**.
- A history of crying, followed by sudden breath-holding in forced expiration with apnea and cyanosis, suggests **cyanotic breath-holding spells**.
- Cyanotic (Tet) spells or breath-holding spells occur commonly after the child wakes in the early morning.

2.4   Cough

- **A cough** is a forceful expiration that can help in the clearance of debris and secretion from the respiratory tract, and it is one of the common presenting complaints in childhood [4].
- **An acute cough** lasts less than 2 weeks and **a subacute cough** lasts 2–4 weeks, while **a persistent or a chronic cough** lasts 4 weeks or more.
- Viral upper respiratory tract infection is the most common cause of cough in children [5].

History Station 2.3: Cough

- **Identity:** Age, address
- **Chief complaint:** Cough
- **History of present illness:**
  1. Onset: Sudden onset with history of choking (foreign body) or a gradual-onset cough
  2. Duration of cough in days: Acute vs. chronic
  3. Timing of the cough: Daytime, nighttime, during sleep, on waking, with exercise
  4. Frequency of cough
  5. Recent history of upper-respiratory tract infection
  6. Cough characteristics: Dry, productive, barking cough, brassy cough (originates from the trachea or large airway), honking, staccato, paroxysmal cough with or without whoop (implies pertussis or parapertussis)
  7. Aggravating factors: Exercise, exposure to tobacco smoke, cold air, respiratory tract infections, exposure to animal dander, dust mites, time of day, position, feeding, seasons that provoke symptoms

Continued on the next page

8. Associated symptoms: Dyspnea, sputum (color, quantity, consistency), hemoptysis, fever, chills, night sweats, weight loss, sore throat, runny nose (may suggest infection), sneezing, noisy breathing (e.g., wheezing and stridor), cyanosis, chest pain, dysphonia (may imply laryngeal or glottic pathology)

- **Past history:**
  A—Birth history: Prematurity, congenital pneumonias, bronchopulmonary dysplasia, or respiratory distress syndrome

  B—Past medical and surgical history: Choking (can be divided into an acute episode, suggesting foreign-body aspiration, or chronic, suggesting incoordinate swallowing), previous attacks of cough, previous hospitalization, diabetes, asthma, immunodeficiency, chronic pulmonary disease, chest trauma, prior radiographs, previous surgeries

- **Medication history:** Response to bronchodilators, antihistamines, antacids or antitussives, recent antibiotic use, ACE inhibitors and B2-antagonists, drug allergies

- **Development history:** Developmental delay or growth retardation

- **Immunizations history:** BCG, DPT, measles, *Haemophilus influenzae* type B (HiB), and pneumococcal vaccine

- **Family history:** Similar symptoms in the family, atopy, asthma, cystic fibrosis, tuberculosis, recurrent infections, and early sibling death

- **Social history:** Tobacco smoke (both passive and active), traveling, exposure to a person with cough or tuberculosis, overcrowded house, school absences, school or day-care attendance, stressors within the family

- **Review of systems:** General state of health, red eyes (conjunctivitis), neuro-muscular weakness, headache (suggests sinusitis), abnormal stools, rectal prolapse, failure to thrive, steatorrhea (cystic fibrosis), vomiting, dysphagia (suggests esophageal foreign body), and itching

Key Points 2.3

- The clinical description of the cough may provide a clue to the etiology: e.g., a barking cough implies **croup**, a brassy cough suggests **a tracheomalacia**, a staccato cough suggests **chlamydia** in infants, choking suggests **foreign-body aspiration**, honking may point to **psychogenic (habit) cough**, while a paroxysmal cough with or without whoop is suggestive of **pertussis** or **parapertussis** and may also point to **cystic fibrosis, asthma**, or **foreign-body aspiration**.

- Nighttime cough suggests **asthma, gastroesophageal reflux (GER)**, or **sinusitis with postnasal drip**.

- Cough associated with fever, chills, night sweats, and weight loss is suggestive of **tuberculosis** or **malignancy**.
- Cough followed by vomiting is typical of **pertussis**.
- Cough with dysphonia may suggest **laryngeal** or **glottic pathology**.
- A cough that disappears during sleep or that is most remarkable when attention is drawn to it is suggestive of **a psychogenic cough**, which most commonly occurs in adolescents [6].
- A cough that occurs during or after eating may suggest **aspiration** or **GER**.

2.5   Wheezing

- **Wheezing** is a continuous musical sound heard mainly during expiration, resulting from partial obstruction of intrathoracic airways [6].
- Although wheezing is usually heard during expiration, it can be heard in both inspiration and expiration when there is fixed airway obstruction in both intra- and extra-thoracic airways [7].
- The word "wheezing" is frequently used imprecisely by parents to describe other noises. Therefore, the use of video clips may be helpful.
- **Viral bronchiolitis** and **asthma** are the most common causes of wheezing in children, so differentiation between these two conditions is mandatory (see Table 2.1) [8].

Table 2.1   Short case scenarios of common causes of wheezing in children [6, 10–12, 90]

Short case scenarios	Diagnosis and special points in favor
A boy, aged 7 years, with a history of atopic dermatitis is referred to the hospital's outpatient department because of a long history of recurrent wheezing, breathing difficulty, and cough. He wakes coughing and wheezing in the early morning, 2 or 3 times a week. The symptoms often occur with exercise and sometimes interfere with sleep. Bronchodilators alleviate the symptoms. According to his mother, he had tended to be wheezy since about 7 months of age. His 4-year-old brother has had eczema since the age of 8 months	**Asthma** – A history of recurrent wheeze, breathing difficulty, and cough – Symptoms often occur with exercise and are improved by bronchodilators. – There is usually a family history of asthma – There is a strong association between asthma and other atopic diseases (e.g., eczema, rhinoconjunctivitis, and food allergy)

Table 2.1 (continued)

Short case scenarios	Diagnosis and special points in favor
A 3-month-old infant presents with wheezing associated with dyspnea, rhinorrhea, sniffles, cough, fast breathing, irritability, poor feeding, and occasional vomiting. The condition deteriorates at night and has been getting worse over the course of 3 days since the onset of symptoms	**Bronchiolitis** – Common age is 1–9 months; it is uncommon after 1 year – The condition deteriorates at night and is getting worse over the course of 3–6 days – Small and premature infants can develop recurrent apnea, which is a serious complication
A 6-year-old unwell child presents with a 6-day history of wheezing, breathing difficulty, fast breathing, cough, chest pain, and fever. In the last day before admission, the condition gets worse. The fever increased and became associated with a rigor as well as brief periods of delirium	**Pneumonia** – The child is usually unwell with cough, fast breathing, fever, and chills – Pleuritic chest pain may be present – The condition usually develops and deteriorates over days
A 2-year-old previously healthy child presents with a 3-day history of wheezing and severe cough, which does not respond to medication. The symptoms developed after sudden choking	**Foreign-body inhalation** – Foreign-body inhalation is common in toddlers – A history of sudden choking or small-object inhalation may present in a previously healthy child – Symptoms do not respond to medication

History Station 2.4: Wheezing

- **Identity:** Age
- **Chief complaint(s):** Wheezing, noisy breathing, or abnormal breathing sound
- **History of present illness:**
1. Onset: Sudden (suggests foreign-body aspiration) or gradual (suggests an infection)
2. Duration: What is the duration of wheezing? Is the wheezing a new presentation or recurrent? Is it episodic or persistent?

Continued on the next page

3. Timing: Nocturnal or early morning wheezing or coughing may suggest GER or sensitivity to common bedroom allergens.
4. Progression and severity of the attack: Compare it to the previous episodes. Does it interfere with the child's activities? Does it awaken the child from sleep?
5. Was the episode of wheezing preceded by choking or gagging?
6. Aggravating and relieving factors: Exercise (asthma), emotions, specific season, cold air, humidity, respiratory infections, feeding (GER and tracheoesophageal fistula (TEF)), agitation or crying (tracheomalacia, bronchomalacia, or a fixed intraluminal or extraluminal obstruction), a certain position. Does the wheezing respond to bronchodilators?
7. Triggering factors: Tobacco smoke, strong odors, fumes, chemicals, dust, animal dander, infection, meals, exercise, change in seasons, or change in temperature or humidity
8. Associated symptoms: Cough (duration in days), sputum, hemoptysis, fever, chest pain, cyanosis, runny nose, sore throat, inability to communicate

- **Past history:**
A—Birth history: Prematurity (bronchopulmonary dysplasia), premature rupture of membranes during birth, mechanical ventilation, or prolonged supplemental oxygen after birth
B—Past medical and surgical history: Previous episodes, history of choking, recurrent chest infections, asthma, congenital heart disease, congestive heart failure, cystic fibrosis, immunodeficiency, allergic rhinitis, food allergies, atopy, results of pulmonary function tests, recent surgical procedures, or intubation
- If there are recurrent attacks of wheezing, ask about age of onset of first attack, triggers, frequency and severity of previous episodes, previous hospitalization, or ICU admissions.
- **Medication history:** Bronchodilators, home nebulizer use, recent use of medications (e.g., beta-blockers, aspirin, and other nonsteroidal anti-inflammatory drugs (NSAIDs)), allergies
- **Developmental history:** Developmental delay, growth retardation
- **Immunization history:** BCG, DPT, and Hib
- **Feeding/dietary history:** Poor feeding, feeding difficulty
- **Family history:** Asthma, wheezing, allergies, hay fever, atopy, and heart disease
- **Social history:** Smoking, traveling, house pets, or overcrowded house
- **Review of systems:** Night sweats; allergy; vomiting; difficulty swallowing; failure to thrive; large, voluminous, foul-smelling, and fatty stools that tend to stick to the toilet (steatorrhea); recurrent/chronic diarrhea; recurrent chest infections

> **Key Points 2.4**
>
> - The presence of wheeze at birth or early infancy suggests **congenital structural abnormalities**.
> - Recurrent episodes of wheezing, cough, dyspnea, and chest tightness are suggestive of **asthma**.
> - In a previously well infant, a new onset of wheezing in combination with symptoms of upper-respiratory tract infection typically points to the diagnosis of **bronchiolitis**.
> - Recurrent wheezing may imply **GER**, particularly if exacerbated by feeding. However, if triggered by upper-respiratory infections, it may point to **reactive airways disease**.
> - Persistent wheezing should lead to a consideration of **mechanical obstruction**, which may have a number of causes (e.g., airway foreign body, external airway compression, or congenital airway narrowing).
> - Recurrent wheezing, especially along with recurrent/chronic diarrhea since early infancy that is difficult to control, should raise the concern for **cystic fibrosis**. Additional probabilities are **primary ciliary dyskinesia**, **recurrent aspiration**, **anatomic abnormalities**, or **immune deficiency**.
> - Wheezing associated with failure to thrive (in spite of good appetite and sufficient dietary consumption), steatorrheic stools, and recurrent infections strongly suggest **cystic fibrosis** [9].

2.6 Stridor

- **Stridor** is a high-pitch, harsh, inspiratory crowing noise, generally caused by acute or chronic obstruction of the airway between the nose and the larger bronchi. It may be heard on expiration if the obstruction is in the subglottic area or trachea, where the sound resembles a wheeze.
- **Acute stridor** is mostly caused by infection (most commonly croup) or upper-airway obstruction, while **chronic stridor** is usually caused by a congenital abnormality (see Table 2.2) [10].

Table 2.2 Short case scenarios of important causes of strider in children [6, 10–12, 90]

Short case scenarios	Diagnosis and special points in favor
A 3-year-old child presents with a crowing noise on inspiration, barking cough, and hoarse voice. The condition was preceded by rhinorrhea, mild cough, sore throat, and low-grade fever for 3 days. The symptoms get worse at night	**Viral croup (laryngotracheobronchitis)** – This typically affects children who are between 6 months and 6 years – It is usually preceded by a common cold lasting 1–3 days – It usually resolves gradually over 1 week

(continued)

Table 2.2 (continued)

Short case scenarios	Diagnosis and special points in favor
A 2-year-old child presents with recurrent attacks of sudden-onset stridor, barking cough, hoarse voice, and respiratory distress. The symptoms are usually worse at night. There are no cold symptoms, and the child is afebrile	**Spasmodic croup** – This usually occurs in children 1–3 years of age – It usually occurs at night – Cold symptoms are often absent and the child has no fever – Attacks are severe and recurrent, but usually last for a short period
A 3-year-old female child presents with acute onset of stridor, sore throat, drooling, high-grade fever, muffled voice, difficulty swallowing, and inability to speak or lie flat. She sits upright with her mouth open and neck extended	**Epiglottitis** – This usually occurs in children 2–7 years old who did not receive Hib vaccine – The cough is usually absent or slight – The child with epiglottitis is usually toxic and unwell
A 4-year-old male child presents with a brassy cough, stridor, respiratory distress, and high fever, preceded by a viral respiratory infection. He does not drool and he is able to lie flat	**Bacterial tracheitis (pseudomembranous croup)** – The usual age is between 3 and 10 years, with a slight male predominance – It is often preceded by a viral respiratory infection
A 1-year-old previously well male child presents with sudden onset of stridor, respiratory distress, and severe cough after a history of choking	**Foreign-body aspiration** – Focal wheeze may be present – There is a history of sudden choking – There is no response to medication
A 2-month-old child presents with intermittent stridor that worsens (or may only be present) on crying, exertion, or lying flat. It is improved by neck extension	**Laryngomalacia** – This is characterized by intermittent stridor that worsens (or may only be present) on crying, exertion, or lying flat – It often develops in the first 6 weeks of life – It often improves with age and resolves at the age of 2 years
A 2-year-old male child presents with stridor, respiratory distress, fever, irritability, drooling, muffled voice, difficulty swallowing, neck pain, and decreased oral intake. The child has a recent history of ear infection	**Retropharyngeal abscess** – This occurs in children aged less than 4 years – About two-thirds of patients have a recent history of throat, ear, or nose infection

History Station 2.5: Stridor

- **Identity:** Age
- **Chief complaint(s):** Crowing noise, noisy breathing, or difficulty breathing
- **History of present illness:**
  1. Onset: Sudden or gradual

Continued on the next page

2. Duration of stridor. Are there recurrent episodes?
3. Timing: Daytime or nighttime
4. Is there any antecedent respiratory infection?
5. Is there a history of choking or playing with any small toys before the episode?
6. Aggravating factors: Increased stridor with stress, agitation, supine position
7. Relieving factors: Rest/sleep, special posture, neck extension (congenital laryngomalacia)
8. Associated symptoms: Respiratory distress, fever (how high is the temperature?), sore throat, voice changes (muffled voice, hoarseness), drooling, cough (barking?), dysphagia, cyanosis, etc.

- **Past history:**
  A—Birth history: Perinatal trauma, method of delivery, forceps delivery, shoulder dystocia, abnormal position in utero, respiratory distress or stridor at birth

  B—Past medical and surgical history: History of choking, history of similar episodes in the past, age of onset of first attack, hemangiomas, trauma or previous surgery, history of intubation (subglottic stenosis)
- **Medication history:** Recent medication use, immunosuppressants, drug allergies
- **Immunization history:** Hib
- **Feeding/dietary history:** Feeding difficulties
- **Family history:** Same symptoms in the family, family history of a recurrent stridor
- **Social history:** Ill contacts, overcrowded house
- **Review of systems:** Headache, malaise, neck swelling, regurgitation, vomiting, diarrhea, or rash

Key Points 2.5

- A sudden onset of stridor with a history of choking should lead to a consideration of **foreign-body inhalation** (particularly in children 6 months to 3 years old) [11, 12].
- Stridor with a history of allergy may suggest **anaphylaxis.**
- Persistent fixed stridor may be caused by **a vascular ring**, or it may infrequently be a result of **vocal-cord paralysis** or **severe micrognathia** (as in Pierre Robin sequence) [11].
- Stridor at rest indicates a severe condition that needs hospital admission [13].

2.7   Chest Pain

- Although chest pain is a common complaint in children—particularly in adolescents—it is an uncommon presentation of cardiac diseases, and it is usually benign and self-limited [14].
- Parents of the child with chest pain are usually anxious and fearful. Therefore, reassurance is necessary, after a thorough history and clinical examination to exclude serious cardiac conditions (see Table 2.3).

Table 2.3 Differentiating features of the various causes of chest pain in children [14, 15, 91, 92]

Diseases or underlying causes	History in favor
Musculoskeletal pain (common)	– Is frequently preceded by a history of unusual effort and physical exertion – Is usually sharp and well-localized – Is reproducible by a specific movement or palpation
Traumatic pain (common) (accidental, abuse)	– Follows or occurs with chest trauma – Is usually localized to the site of trauma
Costochondritis (common) (Tietze syndrome)	– Presents as pain at the costochondral joint – Is more common in teenage females – The pain can be reproduced by palpation of the costochondral joint
Bronchopulmonary pain (common) e.g., asthma, pneumothorax, pneumonia, pleuritis, pleural effusion, and pulmonary embolism	– May be associated with fever, cough, dyspnea, and wheezing or other respiratory symptoms – May worsen with respiration or deep breathing, and may be reproduced by cough – There may be a history of respiratory disorders, such as asthma
Gastroesophageal reflux (common)	– Presents as retrosternal burning pain, which can be diffused – Often occurs after meals (postprandial) – May awaken the patient from sleep and may be associated with a sour taste – Often occurs when the patient lies supine or bends forward and is relieved by antacids
Coronary ischemia, left-ventricular outflow obstruction, coronary anomaly	– Presents as substernal, pressure-like pain – Usually occurs with exertion – Often radiates to the neck, back, or left arm – May be associated with pallor, sweating, palpitation, or syncope
Acute pericarditis (rare)	– Is characterized by acute onset of sharp/stabbing chest pain – May be associated with fever, exacerbated by inspiration, and alleviated by leaning forward, sitting upright, or prone
Myocarditis (rare)	– May present as chest pain with dyspnea, anorexia, and fever – Is usually preceded by a febrile viral illness

Table 2.3 (continued)

Diseases or underlying causes	History in favor
Arrhythmia	– Presents as rapid, forceful beats rather than pain. – May be associated with dizziness or syncope
Psychogenic pain (common)	– Is nonspecific in location and vague in quality – May be associated with family or school stress, other symptoms of anxiety or depression, recurrent somatic symptoms, and trouble sleeping – Disappears during sleep
Idiopathic chest pain (common)	– May present as recurrent chest pain for more than 6 months – Usually occurs at rest – Has no associated symptoms
Hyperventilation (common)	– Is associated with lightheadedness, paresthesia, and underlying anxiety
Precordial catch syndrome (also called Texidor's twinge) (uncommon)	– Is characterized by sudden onset of severe sharp, stabbing pain at left sternal border – Occurs at rest; may be associated with bending or a slouched posture – Lasts seconds to minutes at most – May be increased with breathing; "catches" patient in mid-inspiration
Acute chest syndrome	– Presents as chest pain, fever, shortness of breath, and cough in a patient with sickle-cell disease

History Station 2.6: Chest Pain

- **Identity:** Age, sex
- **Chief complaint:** Chest pain
- **History of present illness:**
  1. Site: Where is it located? Where is the site of maximum severity?
  2. Onset and duration: Sudden onset (foreign body in the esophagus, chest injury should be considered in infants; arrhythmia, chest trauma, and pneumothorax should be considered in older children); gradual onset. How long has the child been having pain? Acute chest pain <2 days (suggests organic cause); chronic chest pain >6 months (suggests psychogenic or idiopathic cause).
  3. Character: What is it like (squeezing, sharp (pericarditis), dull, burning (esophagitis))?
  4. Radiation: Does the pain radiate? If so, where?
  5. Associated symptoms: Fever (may suggest pneumonia, pleuritis, pericarditis, or myocarditis), palpitations, syncope (may suggest arrhythmia or

Continued on the next page

severe anemia), diaphoresis, easy fatigability, cyanosis, pallor, edema, cough, dyspnea, wheezing, heartburn, water brash

6. Time course, pattern, and progression: Does the chest pain follow any pattern? If episodic, ask about duration of attacks. How often does the pain occur (frequency)? If continuous, ask about any changes in severity. Is the pain progressive or regressive?

7. Exacerbating and relieving factors: Exercise (pain that occurs with exercise points to either a cardiac or a respiratory cause), meals, cough, breathing, or movement

8. Severity and relationship of the pain to sleep and activity: Wakes the child from sleep (most likely to be the result of an organic etiology), occurs at rest, or interferes with the child's daily activities (cardiopulmonary cause)

- **Past history:** Exercise tolerance; asthma (increases risk of pneumonia and pneumothorax); recent events: muscle overuse (may suggest musculoskeletal pain), chest trauma, leg trauma (acute chest pain may suggest pulmonary embolism, although rare in children), or recent viral illness; gastroesophageal reflux disease; sickle-cell disease; Kawasaki disease; psychiatric problems; results of prior cardiac and tests (e.g., ECGs or echocardiograms)
- **Medication history:** Recent use of medications, oral contraceptives in adolescent girls (risk of pulmonary embolism), aspirin, steroids, NSAIDs, iron, tetracycline (esophagitis), drug allergies
- **Family history:** Family history of chest pain or sudden unexpected death (may imply hypertrophic cardiomyopathy), cardiorespiratory disease, early coronary artery disease, or stroke in the family, first-degree relatives with congenital heart disease, recurrent syncope, sickle-cell disease, known genetic syndrome (e.g., Marfan or Turner syndromes)
- **Social history:** Stressful life events (e.g., separations, recent bereavement, or serious illness, which suggests psychogenic cause), cocaine, marijuana, or tobacco smoking, impact the pain is having on the child's life, missing school, or social activities.
- **Review of systems:** Abdominal pain, weight loss (tuberculosis), vomiting (gastrointestinal problem)

Key Points 2.6

- A frequent occurrence of chest pain over time is unlikely to be caused by a serious organic pathology [15].
- A family history of early occurrence (<50 years of age) of myocardial infarction, angina, or stroke may suggest **familial hypercholesterolemia, thrombophilia**, and **excessive anxiety**.
- If chest pain is associated with syncope, palpitation, cyanosis, or family history of cardiac arrest, you should consider **cardiac conditions**.
- Sudden death in the family may suggest **cardiomyopathy** or **a familial arrhythmic disorder** [16].

2.8   Syncope

- **Syncope (fainting)** is a temporary and sudden loss of consciousness and postural tone due to *cerebral hypoperfusion*, usually lasting no longer than 1–2 min [17].
- Syncope may be:
  A. **Autonomic** (vasovagal syncope): May *also be referred to as* neurocardio-genic syncope. It is the most common type in children.
  B. **Cardiac**: Mainly related to arrhythmias, but it also can occur due to left-ventricular outflow tract obstruction (e.g., aortic stenosis).
  C. **Noncardiac**: May be due to neurologic etiologies (seizures, migraines), hyperventilation (panic attacks or self-induced), metabolic disturbances (hypoglycemia), or hysteria.

History Station 2.7: Syncope

- **Identity:** Age, sex
- **Chief complaint:** Fainting, blackout, passing out, or transient loss of consciousness
- **History of present illness:**
  1. What was the child doing before the event? What happened immediately before the event? (These questions are helpful in differentiation between syncope and seizure or head trauma.)
  2. Was the event witnessed? What were the exact circumstances surrounding it? Ask about eye movement, respiratory pattern, position of the child during the event, and time spent in this position before the occurrence of syncope.
  3. Duration of loss of consciousness: Typically lasts for 1–2 min; longer duration may suggest a seizure.
  4. The time of day the syncope occurred
  5. Presence of prodromal symptoms: Nausea, headache, warmth, diaphoresis, lightheadedness, palpitations, auditory or visual changes (blurred vision). These symptoms typically last a few seconds before loss of consciousness.
  6. Time since last meal. What did the child eat before the event?
  7. Associated symptoms: Palpitation, chest pain, abnormal movements (can occur in presyncopal period or with syncope), cyanosis, pallor, urinary or fecal incontinence
  8. Were there any residual symptoms after the syncope (e.g., headache or prolonged disorientation)?
  9. Precipitating factors: Hunger, tiredness, fright, exercise (may indicate arrhythmia), standing, heat, recent illness (e.g., upper respiratory infection), or exposure to carbon monoxide (poisoning has symptoms similar to syncope)

Continued on the next page

10. History of head trauma
- **Past history**: Prior episodes of syncope; a history of breath-holding spells (cyanotic or pallid); congenital heart disease; epilepsy; migraine; anemia, or endocrine abnormality (such as diabetes); last menstrual period (possibility of pregnancy in adolescent females)
- **Medication history:** Recent use of medications (e.g., beta-blockers, diuretics, antiarrhythmics, analgesics with sedative properties, or medications that may cause prolonged QT interval (e.g., erythromycin, clarithromycin, amiodarone)), drug allergies
- **Immunization history:** Recent vaccination
- **Feeding/dietary history:** A detailed history of diet, how much the child drinks in a day on average
- **Family history:** Seizure disorders, cardiac disease, sudden death, deafness, Marfan syndrome, hypertrophic cardiomyopathy, prolonged QT syndrome, arrhythmias (particularly at younger ages or requiring pacemaker/implantable defibrillator), breath-holding spells
- **Social history:** Emotional stresses, substance abuse
- **Review of systems:** Vomiting, diarrhea, cough, ear pain

Key Points 2.7

- A family history of sudden death or cardiac disease, palpitations with syncope, or syncope that occurs suddenly and without warning may suggest **a cardiac dysrhythmia**.
- Syncope on standing suggests **orthostatic hypotension**.
- The occurrence of syncope with activity suggests **idiopathic hypertrophic cardiomyopathy**.
- A relatively quick (i.e., a few seconds to 2 min) return to baseline mental status suggests **syncope**, while a delayed return to baseline mental status may suggest **seizures** rather than syncope.
- An anemic child is more liable to have a syncope due to reduced cerebral oxygen delivery [18].

2.9   Sore Throat

- **Sore throat** is throat pain caused by pharyngitis, tonsillitis, or inflammation of the areas that surround the tonsils or the pharynx.
- Sore throat is a very common complaint in children. It is infrequent in the first year of life and is most commonly seen in children aged 5–8 years [19].

- Although sore throat is most commonly a result of **viral** or **bacterial pharyngitis**, it can occur due to other causes, such as epiglottitis, peritonsillar abscess, trauma, or tumors.
- The most common cause of bacterial pharyngitis in children aged >3 years is **group A beta-hemolytic streptococcus (GABHS)**, which is suggested by sore throat associated with high-grade fever, headache, abdominal pain, vomiting, pharyngeal and tonsillar exudate, and tender cervical lymph nodes [19].

History Station 2.8: Sore Throat

- **Identity:** Age
- **Chief complaint:** Sore throat or throat pain on swallowing
- **History of present illness:**
  1. Onset of sore throat
  2. Duration
  3. Associated symptoms: Fever, irritability, cough, runny nose, difficulty breathing, drooling, stridor, voice changes, ear pain, bad breath odor, and oral lesions
  4. History of upper-respiratory tract infection
  5. History of trauma to the throat or neck
  6. Exposure to a foreign body
- **Past history:** Prior streptococcal pharyngitis, rheumatic fever, scarlet fever, previous peritonsillar abscesses, previous episodes of otitis media, chronic sinusitis, pneumonia, diabetes, asthma, immune deficiency, history of tonsillectomy, and history of allergies
- **Medication history:** Recent use of medications (e.g., aspirin, antibiotic, immunosuppressants), drug allergies
- **Immunization history:** DPT, MMR
- **Feeding/dietary history:** Feeding difficulties, poor feeding
- **Family history:** Streptococcal throat infections in the family, similar complaints in household
- **Social history:** Traveling, contact with patient who has a sore throat or upper respiratory tract infection, poor hygiene, exposure to environmental smoke, exposure to irritants, alcohol, oral sexual activity (in sexually active adolescents)
- **Review of systems:** Dysphagia, poor appetite, decreased activity, prolonged fatigue, lymphadenopathy, rash, itchy eyes, red eyes, headache, nausea, vomiting, and abdominal pain

Key Points 2.8

- Sore throat that is associated with upper-respiratory tract infection symptoms (such as cough, runny nose, and conjunctivitis) is suggestive of **viral infection**, the most common cause of sore throat in children [19].
- A scarlatiniform rash and strawberry tongue in a child with sore throat may suggest **scarlet fever**, which is highly suggestive of **group A streptococcal infection**.
- Diagnosis of group A streptococcal infection is very important because it may lead to **rheumatic fever** and **glomerulonephritis**, which are nonsuppurative complications, and **peritonsillar abscess** or **cellulitis** along with **cervical lymphadenitis**, which are suppurative complications of GABHS.
- Fever, painful swallowing, voice changes (such as muffled or "hot potato" voice), drooling, and trismus (a prolonged spasm of the jaw muscles) are suggestive of **peritonsillar abscess** or **cellulitis**.
- A sore throat associated with persistent fever for more than 5 days, red eyes, and skin rash should raise the concern for **Kawasaki disease**.

2.10   Ear Pain

- **Ear pain** can be primary (originates from the ear itself) or secondary (referred from outside the ear). Primary ear pain is commonly caused by **acute otitis media (AOM)** and **otitis externa** [20].
- Diseases of the middle ear are common in infants and toddlers. Otitis externa, infections of the throat, and diseases of the temporomandibular joint are commonly seen in older children and adolescents [21].
- The peak incidence of **acute otitis media** is between 6 and 12 months of life [22].
- Risk factors for acute otitis media can include day-care attendance, tobacco smoke exposure, low socioeconomic status, formula feeding, male sex, winter season, cleft palate, first episode of acute otitis media before 6 months of age, and sibling with recurrent otitis media [23].

History Station 2.9: Ear Pain

- **Identity:** Age, sex
- **Chief complaint:** Ear pain
- **History of present illness:**
  1. Onset, time of onset, and duration: Acute (suggests trauma or infection) vs. chronic
  2. Location of the pain
  3. Quality of pain: Constant vs. intermittent or dull (inflammation) vs. sharp (trauma or neuralgia)

Continued on the next page

4. Severity of pain: Mild, moderate, or severe pain
5. Aggravating or relieving factors: The pain of otitis externa worsens with touching or movement of the ear and during chewing
6. Associated symptoms: Fever (suggests infection), cough, mouth pain, hoarseness of voice (suggests GER), sore throat (suggests referred ear pain), hearing loss, ear discharge, fullness in the ear, tinnitus, vertigo (suggests otogenic pain), multiple somatic complaints (suggests psychogenic ear pain), pruritus of the auditory canal, waking up at night
7. History of upper-respiratory tract infection
8. History of trauma to the ear, foreign body in the ear, or recent history of swimming

- **Past history:** Previous episodes of ear infection (If so, when? How many ear infections has the child had in the past year?), pneumonia, asthma, diabetes, tympanostomy tube placement, cleft palate, Down syndrome, and immune deficiency
- **Medication history:** Immunosuppressants, steroids, antibiotics use (did the child complete the course of prescribed antibiotics?), drug allergies
- **Developmental history:** Is the child's speech development normal?
- **Feeding/dietary history:** Bottle feeding or breastfeeding?
- **Family history:** Large family, family history of otitis media, sibling with recurrent otitis media
- **Social history:** Tobacco smoking (active or passive), recent air travel (may cause ear barotrauma), hobbies (e.g., wrestling may lead to ear trauma), child-care attendance, socioeconomic status
- **Review of systems:** Irritability, lethargy, headache, neck stiffness, anorexia, vomiting, diarrhea, poor feeding

Key Points 2.9

- Mild-to-moderate ear pain of intermittent quality is more likely to be referred from outside the ear [20].
- Breastfeeding is protective against otitis media [22].
- **Acute suppurative otitis media (ASOM)** is a common cause of excessive crying in young children [24].
- Otitis externa can be precipitated by trauma or foreign bodies in the ear [25].
- A history of recent swimming is a common risk factor for otitis externa [21].
- A history of ear pain and fever may suggest **acute otitis media**, especially if it is associated with purulent otorrhea, hearing loss, upper-respiratory tract infection, cough, vomiting, diarrhea, or nonspecific complaints, such as decreased appetite, generalized malaise, lethargy, or irritability.
- Pruritus of the auditory canal, in combination with ear pain that worsens with touching or movement of the ear, is highly suggestive of **otitis externa** [25].
- Persistent ear pain and fever may suggest **acute mastoiditis**.

2.11   Abdominal Pain

- Abdominal pain can originate from intra-abdominal structures (gastrointestinal or non-gastrointestinal causes) or refer from extra-abdominal sites, such as lower-lobe pneumonia, which is also commonly seen in children. It can be **acute** (lasts <2 weeks) or **chronic** (lasts ≥2 weeks) [26].
- **Acute gastroenteritis** is the most common cause of acute abdominal pain in children, while **functional abdominal pain (FAP)** is the most common cause of chronic abdominal pain [27].
- **Acute appendicitis** is the most common surgical cause of the acute abdomen in the pediatric population [26].

History Station 2.10: Abdominal Pain

- **Identity:** Age, sex, address
- **Chief complaint:** Abdominal pain
- **History of present illness:**
  1. Onset
  2. Duration of pain
  3. Location (e.g., right upper-quadrant pain suggests hepatitis, right lower-quadrant pain suggests appendicitis) and radiation
  4. Nature (diffuse, burning, colicky, sharp, dull)
  5. Frequency: If it occurs frequently, ask about the frequency and duration of the episodes.
  6. Timing of pain (nighttime or daytime pain, mealtime, weekends, school days)
  7. Course and progression of pain: Constant or intermittent
  8. Severity of pain: Does it affect the child's activity? Does it wake the child from sleep?
  9. Aggravating and relieving factors: Eating, emesis, defecation, urination, movement, position, respiration, menses, antacids
  10. Associated symptoms: Fever, dyspepsia, nausea, repeated vomiting (undigested food, bilious, blood), diarrhea, constipation, rectal bleeding, melena, anorexia, dysphagia, bloating, distention, jaundice, recurrent oral ulcers, weight loss, weight gain
  11. Characteristics of bowel movement (e.g., any decrease in frequency or change in caliber)
  12. What does the child do when the pain occurs?
- **Past history:** Diabetes, inflammatory bowel disease (IBD), peptic ulcer disease, irritable bowel syndrome (IBS), urolithiasis, celiac disease, migraine, hemolytic anemia, age of menarche (in pubescent female), surgery, endoscopies, X-rays

Continued on the next page

- **Medication history:** Chronic or recent use of medications (e.g., aspirin, NSAIDs, narcotics, oral contraceptives, anticholinergics, laxatives) and drug allergies
- **Developmental history:** Developmental delay, growth retardation
- **Feeding/dietary history:** Change in food consumption, evidence of low fiber diet, spicy food
- **Family history:** Chronic abdominal pain in other family members, IBS, IBD, peptic ulcer disease, celiac disease, urolithiasis, gallstones, migraine, hemolytic anemia
- **Social history:** Recent foreign travel, alcohol, sexual activity, school attendance/sports
- **Review of systems:** Headache, limb pain, dizziness, date of last menstrual period, menorrhagia, vaginal discharge, delayed puberty, stress- or tension-related symptoms, fatigue, weakness, dysuria, hematuria, urinary frequency, chronic cough, wheezing, hoarse voice, sore throat, rash, arthralgia, and symptoms of respiratory tract infection (suggest nonspecific abdominal pain and mesenteric adenitis)

Key Points 2.10

- Radiation of the pain may provide a clue to the diagnosis. For example, the pain of pancreatitis radiates to the back, while the pain of renal stones or a ureteropelvic junction obstruction is radiated to the groin.
- Abdominal pain that is aggravated by defecation suggests **chronic IBD**, while pain that is relieved by defecation suggests **a diagnosis of IBS**.
- The pain of gastroesophageal reflux disease (GERD), gastritis, cholecystitis, or pancreatitis may get worse by eating.
- Abdominal pain occurring at nighttime and relieved by a meal may suggest **peptic ulcer disease** [27].
- Suprapubic or loin pain associated with dysuria, frequency, fever, anorexia, nausea, and vomiting suggests a **urinary tract infection**, a common cause of abdominal pain in children [26].
- Abdominal pain in adolescent females requires special inquiry regarding menstrual history and sexual activity.
- Abdominal pain with fresh bleeding per rectum may suggest **colonic bleeding** or **massive upper-gastrointestinal bleeding**.
- A periumbilical pain that travels to the right lower-quadrant and associates with anorexia, nausea, and vomiting is suggestive of **acute appendicitis**.
- Abdominal pain and vomiting in a child with diabetes mellitus should raise the suspicion of **diabetic ketoacidosis (DKA)**.

2.12 Vomiting

- **Vomiting** is defined as the forceful expulsion of gastric contents through the mouth. It can be divided into three phases: nausea, retching, and emesis. It is not necessary that these phases occur together [28].
- **Nausea** can be defined as the unpleasant and uncomfortable sensation of needing to vomit.
- **Retching** is defined as a coordinated contraction of the abdominal, intercostal muscles and diaphragm against a closed glottis so that there is no expulsion of stomach contents [28].
- Vomiting should be differentiated from **regurgitation**, which is the small, effortless bringing up of one or two mouthfuls of food or stomach content without distress or discomfort.
- Acute vomiting is commonly caused by infection (particularly **viral infection**, such as Norovirus), metabolic conditions, toxic ingestions, or surgical emergencies (e.g., appendicitis or ovarian torsion) [26, 29].

History Station 2.11: Vomiting

- **Identity:** Age, sex, address
- **Chief complaint:** Vomiting
- **History of present illness:**
  1. Duration: Acute (infectious or surgical causes) vs. chronic
  2. Timing: Early morning, daytime, or nighttime
  3. Frequency and course of vomiting
  4. Character and contents (effortless, projectile, bilious, non-bilious, feculent, undigested food, uncurdled milk, bloody, coffee grounds)
  5. Relationship to meals (vomiting of GER or gastric ulcer is relieved by eating a meal)
  6. Associated symptoms: Fever (infectious causes), diarrhea, nausea, abdominal pain, retching, jaundice (suggests hepatitis), pain on swallowing (odynophagia), food refusal, difficulty in swallowing (dysphagia), water brash, unusual odors (suggests a metabolic disorder), constipation, weight loss (suggests systemic disease), failure to thrive, etc.
- **Past history:**
  A—Birth history: Maternal infections, maternal smoking during pregnancy, antenatal ultrasound scan findings, maternal polyhydramnios, prematurity, resuscitation
  B—Past medical and surgical history: Diabetes (suggests DKA), peptic ulcer, CNS disease, contraception, last menstrual period (possibility of pregnancy), urticaria or eczema (suggest food allergy), jaundice, hernia, surgery, upper-GI series, endoscopy

Continued on the next page

- **Medication history:** Recent use of medications, e.g., antibiotics, digoxin, theophylline, chemotherapy, anticholinergics, morphine, ergotamine, oral contraceptives, aspirin (Reye syndrome, aspirin overdose), progesterone, acetaminophen, iron, etc., drug allergies
- **Developmental history:** Developmental delay, vigorous hand or finger sucking, growth retardation
- **Feeding/dietary history:** Type of feeding, feed volume, frequency of feeding, overfeeding, proper formula preparation, effect of any changes in formula, feeding difficulties, ingestion of spoiled food, certain foods that may induce emesis (intolerance to milk, gluten, or soy), food allergy, pica (bezoar)
- **Family history:** Family history of vomiting, surgeries (malrotation, Hirschsprung disease, hiatal hernia,), family history of atopy (food allergy), migraine headaches
- **Social history:** Travel, animal/pet exposure, stresses, emotional disorders, sexual history
- **Review of systems:** Dizziness, lethargy, irritability, seizures, headache (migraine, raised intracranial pressure), vertigo, hearing loss, sweating, rigor, cough (cystic fibrosis, recurrent aspiration, tracheoesophageal fistula), chronic itching, wheezing, apnea, polyuria, dysuria, frequency of micturition, etc.

Key Points 2.11

- Acute vomiting associated with fever that persists for more than 24 h should raise the suspicion of **meningitis**, especially if there is no associated diarrhea [26].
- Persistent vomiting in a neonate or young infant who has no signs of infection may suggest a **congenital gastrointestinal anomaly, CNS abnormality,** or **inborn error of metabolism** [30].
- Bilious vomiting is always pathological (suggests **intestinal obstruction**).
- A sudden onset of bilious vomiting in a previously healthy neonate should lead to a consideration of **malrotation with secondary midgut volvulus,** which needs urgent surgical assessment [29, 30].
- Bilious vomiting with blood in the stool in a sick newborn suggests **necrotizing enterocolitis** [30].
- Vomiting that follows shortly after eating is suggestive of **esophageal** or **gastric outlet obstructions** or **peptic ulcer disease.** However, it may well be **psychogenic,** too [29].
- Vomiting that occurs after ingestion of specific foods may suggest a **food allergy.**
- Persistent, progressive, projectile non-bilious vomiting that occurs immediately after feeding in infants between 2 and 12 weeks of age is suggestive of **pyloric stenosis** [30].

- Effortless vomiting in otherwise well newborns may suggest **GER**.
- Early-morning vomiting may suggest **pregnancy** (in adolescent females) or **increased intracranial pressure (ICP)** (e.g., brain tumor, particularly when there is no nausea).
- Chronic vomiting may suggest **a partial mechanical obstruction** of the gastrointestinal tract (e.g., hiatal hernia) or **a chronic gastrointestinal disease** (e.g., IBD or celiac disease).
- **A ureteropelvic junction (UPJ) obstruction** or **common bile duct stone** can present as vomiting.

2.13   Acute Diarrhea

- **Diarrhea** is defined by the WHO as three or more loose or watery stools per day (or more frequent passage than is normal for the individual) [31].
- **Acute diarrhea** can be defined as a sudden increment in the frequency and water content of stools that <u>resolves within 2 weeks</u>. It is most commonly caused by an infection [31].
- **Rotavirus** is the commonest cause of acute viral gastroenteritis [26].
- The aim of the history is to assess the state of hydration and to find out the etiology of diarrhea (see History Station 2.12 and Table 2.4).

Table 2.4 Differentiating features of the important causative agents of diarrhea in children [10, 26, 32, 90]

Causative agent	History in favor
Rotavirus	– Peak age 3 months to 3 years, common in winter – Foul-smelling, watery diarrhea, vomiting, with or without fever – Preceded by mild upper-respiratory symptoms
Salmonella (salmonellosis)	– Peak age 1 month to 2 years, common in summer, high fever is common – Green, slimy, "rotten egg" odor, and occasionally bloody diarrhea
Shigella (shigellosis)	– Peak age 1–5 years, common in summer – Diarrhea is odorless and watery or bloody with high-grade fever and even seizure
Yersinia enterocolitica	– Peak age 1 month to 2 years, common in winter – Fever with mucoid or bloody diarrhea
Campylobacter jejuni	– Peak age 1–5 years, common in summer – Diarrhea is watery, but it may be bloody, with fever and abdominal cramp
Vibrio cholera (vibriosis)	– Watery, painless diarrhea (resembles rice water) with vomiting and low-grade fever – Does not stop when feeding is discontinued – Occurs during an epidemic
Giardia lamblia (giardiasis)	– Sudden, explosive, watery, foul-smelling diarrhea with bloating, abdominal pain, nausea, and anorexia; fever is rare – Chronic, loose, semisolid diarrhea associated with weight loss, as well
E. histolytica (amebiasis)	– Diarrhea may be mucoid and bloody, with abdominal colic and tenesmus

History Station 2.12: Acute Diarrhea

- **Identity:** Age, sex, address
- **Chief complaint:** Diarrhea, frequent and loose stools <2 weeks
- **History of present illness:**
  1. Onset of diarrhea
  2. Duration and frequency of diarrhea: Number of days of diarrhea and number of stools per 24 h. Ask about the normal stool-passing pattern for the child.
  3. Characteristics of stools (watery, bloody, oily, mucus, mushy, foul odor, formed, explosive)
  4. Relation to eating: Loose motions related to eating (osmotic diarrhea), fasting (secretory diarrhea)
  5. Associated symptoms: Vomiting, fever, abdominal pain or cramps, rectal pain, anorexia, flatulence, weight loss
  6. A history of antecedent mild upper-respiratory symptoms may associate with rotavirus diarrhea.
  7. Season: Rotavirus is common in the winter.
  8. Urine output: Frequency and amount
  9. Fluid and dietary intake
- **Past history:**
  A—Birth history: Low birth weight, prematurity (necrotizing enterocolitis)
  B—Past medical and surgical history: Recent ingestion of spoiled milk, spoiled poultry (*Salmonella*), or seafood (*Vibrio cholera*), immune deficiencies, celiac disease, IBD, otitis media
- **Medication history:** Recent use of medications (e.g., antibiotics, prokinetics, laxatives, immunosuppressants, magnesium-containing antacids, etc.), drug allergies
- **Immunization history:** Rotavirus immunization
- **Feeding/dietary history:** Type of feeding, method of formula preparation, sterilization, type and amount of fluid and solid intake, ingestion of improperly prepared poultry and eggs, food allergies
- **Family history:** Diarrhea in other family members, celiac disease, inflammatory bowel diseases
- **Social history:** Travel, contact with animals/pets, contacts with infected patient, sexual exposures, swimming
- **Review of systems:** Ear pain, cough, dysuria, skin rash, arthralgia, irritability, seizures, and pallor (suggests hemolytic-uremic syndrome)

Key Points 2.12

- Acute diarrhea associated with blood, mucus, and fever may suggest an **enteroinvasive agent**, such as enteroinvasive *Escherichia coli*, *Salmonella* spp. *Shigella* spp., or *Cryptosporidium*.
- Acute diarrhea due to viral infections is commonly seen <u>during the winter</u>, while that due to bacterial infections is more common <u>during the summer</u> [32, 33].
- Diarrhea that occurs abruptly, with no preceding vomiting, is suggestive of **bacterial enteritis** [33].
- Acute diarrhea with fever may point to either **an enteroinvasive pathogen** or **systemic illness** (e.g., meningitis, septicemia, or pneumonia, which can be associated with nonspecific diarrhea) [34].
- Acute diarrhea can be associated with extraintestinal infections (e.g., **otitis media** and **pyelonephritis**).
- Contact with animals can transmit certain pathogens (e.g., *Campylobacter*, *Salmonella*, and *Giardia lamblia*) [33].
- Swimming in dirty water can transmit many bacterial and parasitic agents, especially *Shigella*, *Giardia lamblia*, *Cryptosporidium*, *E. coli* 0157:H7, and *Entamoeba* spp.
- Children who use proton-pump inhibitors or H2 blockers are more susceptible to **bacterial enteritis** [33].
- Children who have recently received antibiotics (e.g., ampicillin) may present with either nonbloody diarrhea (which suggests *C. Difficile* **infection** without colitis or **antibiotic-induced gastroenteritis**) or bloody diarrhea (which suggests **antibiotic-associated pseudomembranous colitis**).
- Acute diarrhea associated with petechial, purpuric rash is suggestive of **Henoch–Schönlein purpura (anaphylactoid purpura)**. In an unwell child, that should raise the concern for **sepsis** [34].
- A child with bloody diarrhea, fatigue, easy bruising, and poor urine output may have **a hemolytic-uremic syndrome (HUS)**.

2.14   Chronic Diarrhea

- **Chronic diarrhea** is the passage of loose and frequent stools <u>for 2 weeks or more</u>, usually secondary to significant malabsorption, as in celiac disease and tropical sprue (see Table 2.5) [34].
- In persistent diarrhea, the cutoff line for the duration is ≥2 weeks, but diarrhea invariably starts as an acute gastroenteritis in an infant.
- **Chronic nonspecific diarrhea** (toddler's diarrhea) is the most common cause of chronic diarrhea in children aged <u>6 months to 3 years</u> who <u>have no failure to thrive</u> [35].

Table 2.5 Short case scenarios of important cases of chronic diarrhea in children [26, 32, 35, 36, 90]

Short case scenarios	Diagnosis and special point(s) in favor
A 2-year-old child presents with a passage of loose stools containing undigested food particles 5 times per day for a duration of 2 months. The symptoms occur during waking hours and become less frequent in the evening. The child is well and has a good appetite and normal growth	**Toddler diarrhea** – Chronic diarrhea commonly occurs in children aged 6 months to 3 years – It involves passage of stools containing undigested food particles about 3–10 times per day
An adolescent male child presents with a 7-month history of passing bloody, mucoid stools associated with fever, tenesmus, weight loss, arthralgia, anorexia, and abdominal pain; the last is exacerbated by defecation	**Inflammatory bowel disease (IBD)** – IBD is more common in older children and adolescents – Crohn's disease is associated with extraintestinal manifestations (e.g., arthralgia and oral or perianal lesions) – Growth failure may occur with or prior to other symptoms
A 1-year-old child presents with a 2-month history of passing loose, mushy, bulky, and smelly stools associated with lethargy, pallor, abdominal distension, and failure to thrive	**Celiac disease** – Symptoms of celiac disease usually appear between 8 and 24 months of age, after gluten introduction
An adolescent male presents with a passage of three to ten stools per day in daytime (not at night). Stooling often occurs after each meal and is associated with a feeling of incomplete evacuation. The child's growth is normal	**Irritable bowel syndrome (IBS)** – The first stool in the morning is usually partially formed and becomes more frequent during the daytime – A feeling of incomplete evacuation is characteristic – Diarrhea may be alternated with constipation
A 9-month-old child presents with a 3-month history of frequent bowel motion associated with vomiting, discomfort on feeding, and squirming. The mother noticed that diarrhea stops when feeding is discontinued. There is a history of acute gastroenteritis preceding the appearance of the symptoms	**Lactose intolerance** – This commonly occurs after acute infection – Diarrhea stops when feeding is discontinued or lactose is restricted – Watery and acidic stools may lead to severe perianal excoriation
A 2-month-old infant presents with a 1-month history of blood-tinged, mucoid diarrhea, starting gradually and associated with vomiting, irritability, poor feeding, and skin rashes. There is a family history of atopy	**Cow's milk protein intolerance** – Symptoms start before the age of 3 months – Diarrhea is chronic and watery or blood-tinged mucoid
A 3-month-old male infant presents with a passage of large, bulky stools with a foul smell for a 1-month duration, associated with failure to thrive. The child has a history of a delayed passage of meconium for >24 h in the neonatal period, and recurrent chest infections over the past 2 months	**Cystic fibrosis** – Newborns may present with meconium ileus – Children may have failure to thrive coupled with voracious appetite, rectal prolapse, and chest infections – There may also be a passage of large, bulky stools with a foul smell secondary to the steatorrhea

History Station 2.13: Chronic Diarrhea

- **Identity:** Age, sex, address, ethnicity/race
- **Chief complaint:** Diarrhea, passage of frequent and loose stools for 2 weeks or more
- **History of present illness:**
  1. Age of onset and duration: When did diarrhea first start? (Immediately at birth? At weaning or after the first exposure to particular foods?)
  2. Frequency and volume of stool output: Number of stools per 24 h. It is important to ask about the normal stool-passing pattern for the child
  3. Ask whether the loose stools are interspersed withnormal ones
  4. Timing of diarrheal episodes: Daytime vs. nocturnal diarrhea (awakening at night to pass stool suggests an organic cause of diarrhea)
  5. Character and consistency of stool: Color, odor, presence of blood (suggests colitis), mucus, or undigested food, greasy, difficult to wash
  6. Aggravating and relieving factors: Stress, effect of eating and fasting on diarrhea
  7. Associated symptoms: Fever, abdominal pain, flatulence, tenesmus, anorexia, nausea, vomiting, hematemesis, melena, hematochezia
- **Past history:**
  A—Birth history: Maternal polyhydramnios (suggests sodium/chloride transporter defect or microvillus inclusion disease), prematurity, necrotizing enterocolitis, pattern of stooling from birth, delayed passage of meconium
  B—Past medical and surgical history: Inflammatory bowel disease (IBD), celiac disease, irritable bowel disease (IBS), constipation, diabetes, hyperthyroidism, a history of gastroenteritis, recurrent pneumonia, intestinal surgery
- **Medication history:** Laxative abuse, recent use of antibiotics, use of magnesium-containing antacids, cholinergic drugs
- **Developmental history:** Developmental delay and growth retardation
- **Feeding/dietary history:** Type of feeding, formula changes, meal preparation, dietary changes and their effect on stool pattern, milk intolerance, (4 "Fs": fiber, fluid, fat, fruit juice), gum (sorbitol), timing and details of weaning
- **Family history:** Family history of chronic diarrhea, consanguinity, celiac disease, IBD, IBS, family history of allergy, milk intolerance
- **Social history:** Travel history, ill contacts, sexual exposure, water supply, and sanitation
- **Review of systems:** Malaise, myalgia, arthralgia, rashes (eczema, perianal irritation are associated with immunodeficiency syndromes), oliguria or anuria, weight loss, or failure to thrive

Key Points 2.13

- A history of chronic diarrhea associated with failure to thrive suggests **malabsorptive conditions** (e.g., cystic fibrosis, celiac disease, and cow's milk protein intolerance) [34].
- Acute exacerbations of chronic diarrhea, especially if associated with fever, is highly suggestive of **inflammatory bowel disease** [34].
- Nocturnal diarrhea should raise the concern for **inflammatory bowel disease** [36].
- **Toddler diarrhea** usually diminishes in frequency in the evening.
- Diarrhea that occurs immediately after birth, with a history of maternal polyhydramnios, is suggestive of **congenital diarrhea** (such as congenital chloride-losing diarrhea) [36].
- Chronic diarrhea that follows an acute gastroenteritis is suggestive of **acquired lactase deficiency**, particularly in certain racial groups (e.g., African Americans and Asians) [26, 32, 36].
- **Osmotic diarrhea** is characterized by a large number of soft stools that are related to eating and that stop after discontinuation of feeding. **Secretory diarrhea** is characterized by a large volume of watery stools that occur even with fasting [32, 37].

2.15   Constipation

- **Constipation** can be defined as a difficult passage of hard, dry stools, commonly associated with a reduction in the frequency of motions to less than 2 stools per week [38, 39].
- The precise definition of constipation may not be as easy as described above in most children. The frequency of bowel movement varies with age; it reduces from more than 4 stools per day in the first week of life to 2 stools per day by 4 months of age and 1 stool per day at 4 years of age. After 4 years, normal frequency of bowel movement varies from 3 per day to 3 per week [38, 39].
- **Functional constipation** is the most common cause of constipation in toddlers [40].

History Station 2.14: Constipation

- **Identity:** Age, sex
- **Chief complaint:** Constipation; hard, dry, difficult-to-pass stools; reduced frequency of motions
- **History of present illness:**
  1. Age of onset and duration of constipation: When did constipation start? Onset after the introduction of weaning suggests celiac disease.
  2. Frequency of stools

Continued on the next page

3. Characteristics of stools (consistency, caliber, and volume of stool): Bulky, fatty stools, foul odor, hard stools, formed or scybalous stools (dry, rabbit-like pellets of small amount), streaks of blood on stool
4. Associated symptoms: Fever, painful defecation (suggests anal fissure), straining, repeated vomiting, abdominal pain or distention, anorexia, soiling (occurs with nerve damage involving the anus or with stool impaction)
5. Transitions: Diapers to toilet training or home to childcare or school (functional constipation)
6. Stool-withholding behavior
7. Water intake

- **Past history:**
  A—Birth history: Maternal diabetes (increased incidence of small left colon), maternal drug intake prior to delivery (opiate, magnesium), prematurity (functional ileus), pattern of stooling from birth, delayed passage of meconium at birth, neonatal complications
  B—Past medical and surgical history: Recent illness, bed rest, fever, celiac disease, cystic fibrosis, eczema, hypothyroidism, diabetes, Hirschsprung disease (congenital megacolon), spinal cord abnormalities, anal fissure, surgery
- **Medication history:** Recent use of medications, e.g., opiates, magnesium, aluminum-containing antacids, iron, antihistamines, anticholinergic agents, etc.
- **Developmental history:** Toilet training (difficult toilet training may associate with encopresis), nocturnal enuresis or daytime wetting, school performance and absence
- **Feeding/dietary history:** Type of feeding, poor feeding, transition from breast to bottle feeding, recent change in diet, excessive cow's milk consumption, contents of diet, low fiber intake
- **Family history:** Family history of constipation, Hirschsprung disease, cystic fibrosis, celiac disease, atopy
- **Social history:** Housing move, sexual abuse, recent birth of a sibling, emotional stress, or family death
- **Review of systems:** Failure to thrive, pallor (celiac disease), unsteady gait (suggests a neuromuscular problem), urinary incontinence or retention, enuresis, urinary tract infection (these urinary conditions are frequently linked to chronic constipation), poor weight gain, respiratory symptoms (cystic fibrosis)

Key Points 2.14

- Stool-withholding behavior with poor dietary and hydration habits is suggestive of **functional constipation**, especially in the absence of alarming symptoms, such as fever, anorexia, weight loss, delayed growth, diarrhea, vomiting, history of delayed passage of meconium, blood in the stool (when an anal fissure is absent), urinary incontinence, or other extraintestinal symptoms [38, 39].
- Severe constipation that starts before 3 years of age should raise the concern of **an organic cause** [39].
- Delayed passage of meconium during the first 24 h of life may suggest **Hirschsprung disease, cystic fibrosis, hypothyroidism, intestinal obstruction**, or **maternal drug use** (e.g., opiates) [38].
- **Hirschsprung disease** should be considered in any child with a history of delayed passage of meconium, enterocolitis in early infancy, constipation before 3 months of age, symptoms of intestinal obstruction (vomiting, abdominal distention), failure to thrive, and trisomy 21 (Down syndrome) with constipation [41].

2.16 Upper-Gastrointestinal Bleeding

- Upper-gastrointestinal bleeding may present as **hematemesis** or **melena**.
- **Hematemesis** is vomiting of blood, which may originate in the esophagus, stomach, or duodenum proximal to the ligament of Treitz. It may be fresh, bright-red blood, or coffee-ground emesis, depending on the duration of the blood exposure to gastric acid [29].
- **Melena** is defined as black, shiny, sticky, foul-smelling stools of tarry consistency, usually resulting from upper-gastrointestinal bleeding above the distal ileum [42].

History Station 2.15: Hematemesis

- **Identity:** Age, sex
- **Chief complaint:** Vomiting blood
- **History of present illness:**
  1. Duration
  2. Frequency of hematemesis
  3. Characteristics of vomitus (coffee-ground material or bright-red blood)
  4. Amount of blood in the vomitus (drops, 1 teaspoonful, 1 tablespoonful)
  5. Forceful retching prior to vomiting blood (Mallory–Weiss tear), recent stress (suggests peptic ulcer or gastritis), or toxic ingestion

Continued on the next page

6. Associated symptoms: Melena, fresh bleeding per rectum, abdominal pain (suggests gastritis, peptic ulcer, or esophagitis), bruising, nosebleeds, weight loss, anorexia, diarrhea, pallor, and jaundice
- **Past history:**
  A—Birth history: Prematurity, nasogastric suctioning, difficult delivery, bleeding during delivery, vitamin K prophylaxis, history of umbilical vein catheterization or infection
  B—Past medical and surgical history: Prior bleeding episodes, a recent history of epistaxis, bleeding disorders, peptic ulcer, gastroesophageal reflux, diabetes, renal failure, liver disease, jaundice, hepatitis, foreign-body ingestion, nasogastric or gastrostomy tube placement, blood transfusion, gastrointestinal surgery, tonsillectomy, adenoidectomy
- **Medication history:** Aspirin, NSAIDs, anticoagulants, steroids, iron, and bismuth (which lead to dark, black stools), acetaminophen, amoxicillin, drug allergies
- **Immunization history:** Hepatitis immunization
- **Feeding/dietary history:** Type of feeding, cracked nipples in a breastfeeding mother, bright-red foods, such as tomatoes, cranberries, beets, red fruit juices, gelatin, and candies
- **Family history:** Same symptoms in the family, peptic ulcer, liver disease, and bleeding disorders, such as von Willebrand disease or hemophilia
- **Social history:** Travel history, alcohol, drug abuse, exposure to hepatitis
- **Review of systems:** Fatigue, disturbed level of consciousness, headache, syncope, palpitation, dyspnea, cough, hemoptysis, hematuria, joint pain

Key Points 2.15

- Coughing of bright-red frothy blood in association with symptoms of respiratory tract infection is suggestive of **hemoptysis** rather than **hematemesis** [29].
- Hematemesis may occur due to **Mallory–Weiss tears, esophagitis, esophageal varices, peptic ulcers, gastritis, iron ingestion, vascular malformations**, or **bleeding disorders**.
- Ingestion of maternal blood from cracked nipples is a common cause of hematemesis in breastfed neonates [29, 36].
- **Prematurity** and **difficult delivery** increase the risk of gastric ulcerations and erosions that may bleed [42].
- Hematemesis preceded by prolonged, forceful retching or vomiting in a previously well child suggests **Mallory–Weiss syndrome**, which occurs due to tears in the lower esophagus or stomach [36].

- Hematemesis can result from an extraintestinal source, such as swallowing blood that originates from the upper respiratory tract (e.g., **post-tonsillectomy** and **adenoidectomy** bleeding or **epistaxis**) [36].
- Sometimes certain drugs, foods, or food-coloring agents can mimic blood.
- The persistence of an unrecognized esophageal foreign body may cause esophageal edema and erosion, which may result in hematemesis [42].

2.17   Lower-Gastrointestinal Bleeding

- Lower-gastrointestinal tract bleeding is bleeding from the gastrointestinal tract distal to the ligament of Treitz.
- **Hematochezia** can be defined as the passage of bright-red or maroon-colored blood per rectum. It usually indicates lower-gastrointestinal bleeding or, rarely, may occur due to massive bleeding above the distal ileum [43].
- **Currant-jelly stools** are gelatinous stools composed of a mixture of sloughed mucosa, blood, and mucus, usually indicating **intussusception** [43].

History Station 2.16: Lower-Gastrointestinal Bleeding

- **Identity:** Age, sex
- **Chief complaint:** Anal bleeding, rectal bleeding, presence of blood in stool
- **History of present illness:**
  1. Duration
  2. Stool characteristics: Bright red, dark red, melena, currant-jelly, fecal mucus
  3. Location of blood in relation to the stool: Is the blood mixed in the stool (suggests colitis), coating the outside of the stool (suggests anal fissure), or occurring just after defecation?
  4. Quantity and severity of bleeding
  5. Consistency of the accompanying stool: Diarrhea suggests colitis; hard stool suggests anal fissure
  6. Any changes in bowel habits or stool caliber
  7. Associated symptoms: Diarrhea, abdominal pain (suggests colitis, IBD, or intussusception), constipation, anorectal pain (suggests anal fissure), perianal lesions, vomiting, hematemesis, tenesmus, excessive straining during defecation, anorexia, jaundice, weight loss, mouth sores, fever, malaise
- **Past history**:
  A—Birth history: Maternal drug use (e.g., warfarin, anticonvulsants, isoniazid, rifampicin), mode of delivery, low birth weight, prematurity (necrotizing enterocolitis), neonatal jaundice, vitamin K prophylaxis

Continued on the next page

B—Past medical and surgical history: Same attack in the past, inflammatory bowel disease, constipation, anorectal conditions, peptic ulcer, hepatitis, jaundice, liver disease, blood transfusion, previous or recent gastrointestinal surgery, recent investigations

- **Medication history:** Anticoagulants, aspirin, NSAIDs, steroids, drug allergies
- **Feeding/dietary history:** Bright-red foods and drinks, cow's milk, soy formula, ingestion of uncooked meat
- **Family history:** Liver disease, peptic ulcer, anorectal conditions, inflammatory bowel disease, bleeding disorders (e.g., von Willebrand disease or hemophilia)
- **Social history:** History of travels, sexual abuse
- **Review of systems:** Disturbed level of consciousness, headache, syncope, palpitation, dyspnea, fatigue, arthralgia (suggests IBD), skin lesions, epistaxis, hematuria, pallor

Key Points 2.16

- A sudden onset of severe, episodic abdominal pain associated with vomiting and passage of currant-jelly stools in the first 2 years of life should raise the concern for **intussusception**, which is frequently preceded by an upper-respiratory infection [33, 43].
- The most common cause of bleeding per rectum in children is **acute anal fissure** [44].
- Streaks of bright-red blood on the outside of the stool may suggest a diagnosis of **anal fissure**, particularly if associated with the passage of hard, painful stools [36, 44].
- In a young child, recurrent passage of small amounts of blood in the stool without pain may suggest **a juvenile polyp**, especially when there is no history of constipation [36, 43].
- The occurrence of bleeding per rectum in conjunction with diarrhea and abdominal pain is suggestive of **an infectious colitis** or **inflammatory bowel disease**, while bleeding per rectum in the absence of diarrhea or pain may suggest **proctitis** [36].
- Rectal bleeding in **ulcerative colitis** is usually profuse, with tenesmus and hypogastric pain [45].
- Children with **Crohn's disease** may present with right-iliac fossa pain, weight loss, failure to thrive, and perianal disease [45].
- In early childhood (<7 years of age), acute onset of colicky abdominal pain, polyarthritis, hematuria, purpura, vomiting, and rectal bleeding should raise the possibility of **Henoch–Schönlein purpura (HSP)**, particularly if preceded by a viral illness [36, 42, 43].

2.18   Jaundice

- **Jaundice** is a yellowish discoloration of the skin, sclerae, and mucous membranes, resulting from elevated levels of serum bilirubin, a byproduct of the breakdown of heme proteins [46].
- It can result from conjugated hyperbilirubinemia, which occurs secondary to cholestatic conditions or direct hepatocellular injury (it is always pathologic), or from unconjugated hyperbilirubinemia, which occurs secondary to overproduction of bilirubin, impaired conjugation, or impaired uptake of bilirubin by hepatocytes [47].
- Although many causes of jaundice are pathologic, physiologic benign jaundice in neonates is the most common clinically encountered jaundice in pediatrics; it affects roughly more than half of newborns in the first week of life [47].

History Station 2.17: Jaundice

- **Identity:** Age, sex, address, ethnicity/race
- **Chief complaint:** Jaundice, yellowish discoloration of the skin and whites of the eyes
- **History of present illness:**
  1. Time of onset and duration of jaundice: When was jaundice first noticed? On which day of life (in neonates)?
  2. Distribution and progression: Gradual development of jaundice that progresses caudally may suggest physiologic jaundice or breastfeeding jaundice.
  3. Are there any prodromal symptoms?
  4. Associated symptoms: Fever (suggests infection), abdominal pain, anorexia, vomiting, hematemesis, melena, diarrhea, constipation, weight loss, unexplained itching (suggests cholestatic liver disease), failure to thrive
  5. Color of stool and urine: The passage of dark urine and pale/light-colored stools suggests cholestasis.
- **Past history:**
  A—Birth history: Course of the pregnancy, maternal infections and illnesses, medications used during the pregnancy, gestational diabetes, intrauterine growth restriction, prematurity, low birth weight, delayed clamping of the umbilical cord, irritability, newborn hypoglycemia, inability to pass meconium, history of neonatal jaundice, jaundice during the first 24 h of life, vitamin K deficiency with bleeding, or birth trauma
  B—Past medical and surgical history: History of previous jaundice, history of exposure to blood or blood products, chronic liver diseases, hemolytic anemia, autoimmune disease, ulcerative colitis (risk of sclerosing cholangitis), hepatitis serology, liver function tests, liver biopsy, or previous biliary surgery

Continued on the next page

- **Medication history:** Recent introduction of medications (e.g., antibiotics, acetaminophen (paracetamol), isoniazid, phenytoin, etc.), drug allergies
- **Immunization history:** Hepatitis immunization
- **Feeding/dietary history:** On breastfeeding or bottle feeding, bean ingestion, shellfish ingestion (hepatitis)
- **Family history:** Consanguinity, family history of unexplained liver disease (suggests Wilson disease or another genetic cause), autoimmune disease (type 1 diabetes, celiac disease, hypothyroidism), hemolytic disorders, familial jaundice, history of perinatal infant death (metabolic disorders), lung disease, alpha1-antitrypsin deficiency, other member of the family affected, sibling with neonatal jaundice required phototherapy, and blood-group incompatibility between the parents
- **Social history:** History of foreign travel, IV drug abuse, exposure to hepatitis, social stress, alcohol, poor school performance, or change in mental status and/or handwriting (suggests Wilson disease)
- **Review of systems:** Change in mental status, slurring of words (may suggest Wilson disease), lethargy, irritability, poor feeding, arthralgia, pruritus, rash, bruising, or pallor

Key Points 2.17

- Rapid progression and early occurrence (in the first 24 h of life) of jaundice and jaundice that occurs or persists beyond 2 weeks of age suggest **a pathological etiology** [48].
- Jaundice in a child with a past history or family history of a blood disorder suggests **hemolysis** [46].
- In the neonatal period, cephalocaudal progression of jaundice usually correlates with the elevated levels of serum bilirubin [49].
- Jaundice that is preceded by prodromal symptoms is suggestive of an **infectious etiology** [46].
- Jaundice in a healthy neonate on the second or third day of life suggests **physiological jaundice**, particularly when there are no pale stools or dark urine [36].
- Lethargy, hypotonia, irritability, and poor feeding in jaundiced infants indicate severe hyperbilirubinemia, which can progress to **kernicterus** [49].
- Jaundice that occurs in conjunction with symptoms of chronic illness (e.g., weight loss or pruritus) should raise the possibility of an **inflammatory** or **metabolic process**.
- The occurrence of jaundice, hematemesis, melena, and a change in mental status (sensorium) in the child should lead to a consideration of **progressive** or **fulminant hepatic failure** [46].

2.19 Hematuria

- **Hematuria** is the presence of red blood cells (RBCs) in the urine. It is either gross or microscopic (>5 RBCs per high-power field seen on microscopy of centrifuged urine). It can result from glomerular causes or non-glomerular causes, the latter being more common [50, 51].

History Station 2.18: Hematuria

- **Identity:** Age, sex, address
- **Chief complaint:** Passage of bloody urine, red-colored urine, or the presence of blood in the urine
- **History of present illness:**
  1. Duration
  2. Timing of hematuria: Initial (urethral source), constant (glomerular or renal source), or terminal (trigonitis or hemorrhagic cystitis)
  3. Color of urine: Red or pink (lower urinary tract origin), tea- or cola-colored (renal or glomerular)
  4. Intermittent or persistent: Does hematuria occur with each passage of urine?
  5. Associated symptoms: Fever (suggests infectious or systemic illness); flank pain (renal colic suggests a stone); suprapubic pain; perineal or abdominal pain; incontinence; dysuria, frequency, urgency, or voiding symptoms (may suggest bacterial or viral hemorrhagic cystitis)
  6. Precipitating factors: Recent trauma (to trunk, abdomen, or perineum), Foley's catheterization, or strenuous exercise
  7. Stone, tissue or clot passage in urine
  8. Concurrent upper respiratory infection or gastroenteritis (suggests IgA nephropathy)
  9. Drops of blood or spotting in underwear between or after voiding (suggests bleeding from urethra in prepubertal boys or non-urethral sources of bleeding, such as perineal or vaginal bleeding in females)
  10. Decreased fluid intake
- **Past history**: Previous episodes of gross hematuria or UTI; recurrent upper-respiratory illness, recent sore throat (group A streptococcus), impetigo (may suggest post-infectious glomerulonephritis); bloody diarrhea; coagulopathy; sickle-cell disease/trait; G6PD deficiency; history of renal stone; recent abdominal surgery or trauma; previous investigations
- **Medication history:** Recent use of medications (e.g., heparin, warfarin, aspirin, ibuprofen, rifampin, nitrofurantoin, naproxen, phenobarbital, phenytoin, cyclophosphamide, etc.), drug allergies
- **Feeding/dietary history:** Type of feeding, ingestion of beetroot, fava beans, berries, rhubarb, or food coloring
- **Family history:** Hematuria, renal diseases, renal failure (may suggest hereditary nephritis or cystic disease), renal stone (suggests renal stone, hypercal-

Continued on the next page

ciuria, or metabolic disease), systemic lupus erythematosus (SLE), polycystic kidney disease, coagulation disorders, sickle-cell disease/trait (suggests sickle nephropathy, papillary necrosis, or hemoglobinuria), hypertension, premature deafness (Alport syndrome)

- **Social history:** Child abuse, exposure to hepatitis B or C, occupational exposure to toxins
- **Review of systems:** Mental status changes, headache, visual changes (diplopia), pallor, syncope, palpitation, dyspnea, diarrhea, edema, rashes and joint pain (suggests systemic illness or immunologic-mediated process), heavy menses, epistaxis, or bleeding from any other source, e.g., gums or gastrointestinal bleeding (suggests coagulopathy)

Key Points 2.18

- Passage of bright-red- or pink-colored urine or visible blood clots suggests **urinary tract bleeding**, while passage of brown-, tea-, or cola-colored urine suggests **renal** or **glomerular bleeding** [50, 51].
- The combination of gross hematuria, facial or body edema, hypertension, and decreased urine output may suggest **glomerulonephritis**, e.g., acute post-streptococcal glomerulonephritis (APSGN) or IgA nephropathy [50].
- Passage of bloody urine only at initiation of micturition suggests **urethral bleeding**, whereas terminal hematuria suggests **trigonitis** or **hemorrhagic cystitis**, and a constant bloody stream indicates **a renal source** [51].
- Hematuria that is preceded by an upper-respiratory infection or, in some cases, gastroenteritis, or an episode of impetigo may suggest **acute post-streptococcal glomerulonephritis, hemolytic-uremic syndrome (HUS)**, or **Henoch–Schönlein purpura nephritis** [50].
- **IgA nephropathy** (Berger disease) commonly presents with recurrent episodes of microscopic or frank hematuria, which is often preceded by a viral prodrome 1–3 days before the onset of hematuria [50].
- Hematuria associated with dysuria, fever, frequency, or urgency suggests **a urinary tract infection**.
- Gross hematuria with renal colic that may radiate to the groin is suggestive of **renal stone disease**.
- Painless hematuria may point to **a glomerular origin** [51].
- Rashes and joint pain may suggest **Henoch–Schönlein purpura nephritis** or **SLE nephritis**.
- An abdominal mass, with or without abdominal pain, should raise the concern for **Wilms tumor**, which may be associated with microscopic hematuria in 50% of cases, whereas gross hematuria is uncommon.
- The occurrence of hematuria in conjunction with a change in mental status, headache, visual changes (diplopia), epistaxis, or heart failure is suggestive of **significant hypertension** [52].

2.20 Edema

- **Edema** is a clinical condition characterized by either a generalized or localized accumulation of excessive fluid in the interstitial space of the body, resulting in swelling of the tissue. It may be secondary to albumin deficiency, lymphatic or venous vessels obstruction, or trauma [53, 54].

History Station 2.19: Edema

- **Identity:** Age, sex
- **Chief complaint(s):** Swollen ankles and feet, periorbital swelling, body swelling
- **History of present illness:**
  1. Onset of the edema: Sudden or gradual onset
  2. Duration and time course of the edema: Congenital or started later on (ask about child's age at time of onset)
  3. Timing: Does the swelling increase or decrease at certain times during the day?
  4. Character, location, and progression of edema: Is it localized or generalized? Where does it start: the ankles, the abdomen, or the periorbital region? Weight gain, difficulty putting shoes on, and tight-fitting clothes (suggests generalized edema)
  5. Intermittent or persistent swelling
  6. Associated symptoms: Fever, pain, decreased urine output, bloody urine (smoky or red), flank pain, dyspnea (ascites, pleural effusions, or pulmonary edema), or distress (determine urgency of treatment)
  7. History of insect bite, trauma, or burn
- **Past history:**
  A—Birth history: Maternal nutrition, neonatal hemolytic disease, neonatal problems that may indicate possible renal damage
  B—Past medical and surgical history: Renal disease, heart disease, gastrointestinal disease, liver disease, menstrual cycle problems, premenstrual bloating, pregnancy (in adolescent females), skin rash, recent pharyngitis or impetigo, sickle-cell disease, venous catheters, malignancies, urinary tract infection, previous urinalysis (may help date the onset of the edema)
- **Medication history:** Current medications and allergies; over-the-counter drugs; corticosteroid; lithium; oral contraceptives; estrogen; antihypertensives: ACE inhibitors, diuretics, and vasodilators (calcium channel blockers, minoxidil)
- **Feeding/dietary history:** Poor feeding, feeding difficulties, poor protein intake (kwashiorkor), allergic reactions to foods (cow's milk), excess salt intake in diet (may contribute to edema), and dietary changes

Continued on the next page

- **Family history:** Renal diseases, cystic fibrosis, lupus erythematosus, deafness, Alport syndrome, recurrent angioedema, liver disease, diabetes mellitus, autoimmune disorders, and heart disease
- **Social history:** Risk of malnutrition, exposures to toxins, alcohol, chemicals, sexual activity, prenatal exposures to hepatitis B, or HIV
- **Review of systems:** Itching, cough, diaphoresis, poor exercise tolerance, anorexia, chronic diarrhea (protein-losing enteropathy or lymphatic obstruction), jaundice, bleeding per rectum, mouth ulcer, failure to thrive, fatigue, irritability, restlessness, rash, and joint pain (suggests collagen vascular disease)

Key Points 2.19

- Determination of the time course of the edema is very important for differentiating between an acquired condition and a congenital condition [53].
- Pedal edema in the newborn suggests **Turner syndrome**.
- A history of a progressive, generalized edema, including a marked periorbital edema, but with minimal systemic complaints, is suggestive of **nephrotic syndrome** [53].
- A history of streptococcal infection 1–3 weeks prior to the onset of either generalized or facial edema, associated with cola-colored urine, is strongly suggestive of **post-streptococcal glomerulonephritis** [53].
- A history of edema, poor appetite, and growth failure is suggestive of **chronic renal failure**.
- The presence of edema in conjunction with jaundice, steatorrhea, failure to thrive, or abdominal pain may suggest a diagnosis of **chronic liver disease** or **protein-losing enteropathy**.
- Localized edema in a child with sickle-cell disease, congenital heart disease, venous catheters, or malignancies should raise the concern for venous thrombosis.
- Although **allergic reaction, infection, and trauma** are the most common causes of localized edema, it can also be caused by diseases of the lymphatic system, as well as by venous obstruction [54].

2.21 Polyuria and Urinary Frequency

- **Polyuria** can be defined as urine output of 2 L/m^2 or more over 24 h [55].
- The most important differential diagnoses for polyuria and polydipsia are **diabetes mellitus**, **diabetes insipidus** (central or nephrogenic), and **primary polydipsia** [55].

History Station 2.20: Polyuria and Urinary Frequency

- **Identity:** Age, sex
- **Chief complaint(s):** Excessive urination, excessive urinary frequency or volume, or bedwetting
- **History of present illness:**
  1. Onset: Abrupt onset (as in central diabetes insipidus) or gradual onset (like excessive water intake)
  2. Duration
  3. The number of daytime voids and nighttime voids, nocturnal enuresis
  4. Associated symptoms: Polydipsia (excessive fluid intake), nocturia, incontinence, daytime and nighttime enuresis, urgency, poor urinary stream, dysuria, straining to urinate, persistent dribbling of urine, abdominal and perineal pain, or fever
  5. Waking at night to drink or constant daytime thirst
- **Past history**: Age of onset of excessive urination, history of diabetes, sickle-cell anemia, renal disease (acute or chronic renal failure, polycystic kidney disease, recurrent urinary tract infections, history of urinary tract obstruction), malignancy, hypercalcemia, dehydration, CNS infection, history of head trauma or surgery
- **Medication history:** Recently taken medications (e.g., diuretics, lithium, antibiotics (such as demeclocycline), antifungals, antivirals, or antineoplastic agents), drug allergies
- **Developmental history:** Age of toilet training and growth pattern (growth failure is a feature common to both central and nephrogenic diabetes insipidus)
- **Feeding/dietary history:** Type of feeding, volume of milk intake, fluid intake diary
- **Family history:** Family members with polydipsia, polyuria, genitourinary disorders; parental age of toilet training, infants with poor growth, early infant deaths, sickle-cell disease, or diabetes
- **Social history:** Sexual abuse, stressful conditions
- **Review of systems:** Headache, visual disturbances, irritability, gait disturbances, lower-extremity weakness, back pain, leg pain, polyphagia, vomiting, constipation, or involuntary defecation

Key Points 2.20

- The sudden onset of polyuria, polydipsia, and nocturia, with a desire for iced water, may suggest **central diabetes insipidus** [56].
- Polyuria may present after the first year of life in **familial central diabetes insipidus** (which is usually an autosomal dominant disease) [55].

- Polyuria associated with headache or visual disturbances may suggest **CNS tumors** [56].
- In the first weeks of life, a profound polyuria, lethargy, vomiting, poor weight gain, hypernatremic dehydration, or unexplained fever should raise the possibility of **inherited nephrogenic diabetes insipidus** [55, 56].
- **Primary polydipsia** (also called psychogenic polydipsia) is clinically difficult to differentiate from **diabetes insipidus**, as symptoms of primary polydipsia are similar to those seen in diabetes insipidus, although there may be no nocturia or predilection for cold water or ice [56].
- **Sickle-cell disease** may cause water diuresis, due to renal infarction [37].

2.22   Diabetic Ketoacidosis

- **Diabetic ketoacidosis (DKA)** is a condition that occurs in children with diabetes mellitus, due to severe insulin deficiency or insulin inefficiency. Although generally resulting from omitted insulin injections, stressful conditions, or unsuccessfully managed intercurrent illness in a child with type 1 diabetes, it can occur in about 20–45% of children with new-onset diabetes [57].
- The criteria for diagnosis of diabetic ketoacidosis (DKA) include blood sugar ≥ 200 mg/dL, pH < 7.3, or bicarbonate <15 mEq/L, ketosis (presence of ketones in the blood, urine, or both) [57].

History Station 2.21: Diabetic Ketoacidosis

- **Identity:** Age
- **Chief complaint(s):** Nausea, vomiting, abdominal pain, fatigue, excessive urination, excessive fluid intake, fast breathing and air hunger, headache, drowsiness, and coma
- **History of present illness:**
  1. Duration of the symptoms
  2. Initial level of blood glucose and ketones
  3. Fruity smell on the breath
  4. History of weight loss, nocturia, nocturnal enuresis, polyuria, polydipsia, or polyphagia
  5. Precipitating factors: Noncompliance with insulin, trauma, surgery, psychological stress, exercise, infection, intercurrent illness, and pregnancy

Continued on the next page

- **Past history**: New onset of diabetes, age of onset of diabetes, initial manifestations, initial investigations, hospitalizations (date, cause, duration, progression of the condition, frequency of hospitalizations), patient condition between the attacks, self-monitoring of blood glucose (frequency, results in book/device memory), polycystic ovary syndrome, recurrent infections, renal disease, autoimmune thyroiditis, celiac disease, Addison disease, vitiligo, or other autoimmune diseases
- **Medication history:** Details of insulin therapy (route–pump/injections, dose, frequency, timing, sites, and adjustment for blood glucose), recently taken medications, drug allergies
- **Developmental history:** Developmental delay, school progress, growth delay
- **Feeding/dietary history:** High-calorie diet, excessive eating
- **Family history:** Family functioning/coping, diabetes, thyroid disease, celiac disease, or other autoimmune diseases in the family
- **Social history**: Psychological stress, severe emotional upset, smoking/drinking
- **Review of systems:** Headache, behavioral change with restlessness, drowsiness, seizures, dyspnea, blurred vision, air hunger, decreased urine output, sunken eyes, cough, nausea, vomiting, abdominal pain, ear pain (otitis media), fever, dysuria (urinary tract infection), obesity, depression, etc.

Key Points 2.21

- A child with DKA can present with a variety of symptoms, depending on the severity of the condition and the age of the child.
- Older children may present with **polyuria**, which occurs in spite of a state of clinical dehydration, due to the glucose-induced osmotic diuresis. This can help to differentiate patients with DKA from patients with gastrointestinal disorders (e.g., gastroenteritis). Other symptoms are **polydipsia**; **fatigue**; **nausea**; **vomiting**; **abdominal pain**; **deep-sighing respirations (Kussmaul breathing)**, with **acetone odor**; and **somnolence** or a **disturbed level of consciousness** [58].
- In infants, **decreased activity, irritability, weight loss, and dehydration** may be the presenting symptoms of DKA [58].
- Duration of symptoms varies with age; it may be days in toddlers or months in adolescents [59].
- **Weight loss** in a child with DKA may be due to dehydration and loss of calories [59].
- In a child with DKA, a history of severe headache or any decrement in consciousness level should raise the concern for **cerebral edema**.

2.23   Failure to Thrive

- **Failure to thrive (FTT)** is a symptom of an underlying cause, not a diagnosis on its own. It is usually seen in a child younger than 5 years of age whose physical growth is significantly less than that of his/her peers [60, 61].
- It can be divided into:
  - **Nonorganic FTT:** Poor growth without a medical cause. It is usually linked to poverty or poor interaction between the child and his/her caregiver.
  - **Organic FTT:** Occurs due to an underlying medical pathology, e.g., inflammatory bowel disease or congenital heart disease [60].

History Station 2.22: Failure to Thrive

- **Identity:** Age, sex, address, ethnicity/race
- **Chief complaint:** Inadequate growth
- **History of present illness:**
  1. Onset and duration: When did the parents become concerned about the problem? (Record the exact date.)
  2. Child's pattern of growth over time
  3. Aspects of growth that have been affected; which domain was affected first?
  4. Associated symptoms: Change in appetite, weight loss, fever, vomiting, abdominal pain, diarrhea, steatorrheic stools, or constipation
- **Past history:**
  A—Birth history: A history of abortions, either spontaneous or therapeutic. Was the infant wanted? Number of previous pregnancies, antenatal care, maternal infection, maternal diet during pregnancy, maternal illness, hypertension or preeclampsia, depression, radiation exposure, maternal drug use (Which drugs did she use?), herbal supplements, tobacco, alcohol, intrauterine growth restriction, prematurity, low birth weight, prenatal insult, perinatal illnesses, neonatal jaundice, and malformations or chromosomal anomalies
  B—Past medical and surgical history: Previous hospitalizations; previous illnesses (e.g., gastroenteritis, recurrent pneumonia); chronic diseases (diabetes, hyperthyroidism, inflammatory bowel disease, celiac disease, renal disease, congenital heart conditions, neurologic disorders, immunodeficiency); previous surgeries; and previous investigations
- **Medication history:** Chronic use of medications, chemotherapy
- **Developmental history:** Loss (regression) of developmental milestones or developmental delay
- **Feeding/dietary history:**
  - **For an infant**: Type of feeding (breast or formula feeding)
  - If **a breastfed infant**, then ask about the number of feedings per day, the duration of each feeding, satisfaction of the mother and the baby, voiding,

Continued on the next page

vomiting, and stooling. These should all be recorded. Also record the baby's sleep pattern, feeding difficulties (such as poor sucking and swallowing), fatigue during feeding, and lactation failure.

- If **a formula-fed infant**, then ask about the type of milk used (commercial or homemade formula), details of the formula preparation, and by whom it is prepared. The mixing process (to ensure appropriate dilution) should be reviewed (as adding too much water to powdered formula results in inadequate nutrition). Also, the number of ounces that the baby takes in a 24-h period and the number of diapers wet per day (6–8 diapers) should be recorded. Consider observing a feeding. This can be done while taking the history.

- **For an older child**: Ask about the time of the introduction of semisolids and solids. The quantity and type of foods and juices consumed should be noted. Parental dietary restrictions (e.g., low fat), dietary restrictions because of food allergies, and the timing and duration of meals should be noted. Where does the child eat each meal and with whom? Are distractions (television or video games) present during meals? Is the child a picky eater? If this information proves difficult to elicit, the parents can be sent home with a nutritional diary to fill out prospectively and bring in at the next visit.

- **Family history:** Consanguinity, the ages at which the parents achieved puberty, parental heights and weights, biologically related siblings with poor growth, short stature in the family, deaths of siblings or relatives during early childhood (metabolic or immunologic disorders), cystic fibrosis

- **Social history:** Parental histories of abuse or neglect in childhood, parental substance abuse, parental depression, current stresses, recent travel, financial difficulties, family income, marital discord, the child's living arrangements (including primary and secondary caregivers), housing, the family's social supports, parents' educational levels, child-care attendance, or homelessness

- **Review of systems**: Polyuria, polydipsia, jaundice, cough, snoring or mouth breathing, cyanosis, polyphagia, irritability, skin rash, arthritis, weakness, diaphoresis or fatigue while eating, poor sucking, swallowing difficulties

Key Points 2.22

- Knowing the growth domain that is affected first may provide clues for the etiology. For example, the child's weight is affected first and most severely in acquired conditions, followed by the length, and lastly the head circumference. In congenital, endocrinal, or genetic conditions, all growth domains may be affected symmetrically [61].

- Maternal hypertension or preeclampsia may result in a small for a gestational-age baby [62].

- Although the infant of a diabetic mother may have macrosomia, he/she may fail to gain weight due to postnatal cardiac complications [62].

2.24   Headache

- **Headache** is a common complaint in pediatrics, especially in older children and adolescents [63, 64].
- It can be classified into:
    - **Primary headaches** are often recurrent and episodic (e.g., migraine, tension-type, and cluster headaches). There is no underlying cause.
    - **Secondary headaches** are a symptom of an underlying intracranial or medical condition (e.g., tumor or trauma) (see Table 2.6) [64].
- Headaches may also be classified in terms of time course, into:
    - **Acute headache** (e.g., intracranial hemorrhage, infections: meningitis, sinusitis, pharyngitis, otitis media)
    - **Acute recurrent headache** (e.g., migraine, cluster headache, or hypertension)
    - **Chronic progressive headache** (e.g., neoplasm, abscess, hydrocephalus, pseudotumor cerebri)
    - **Chronic nonprogressive headache** (e.g., tension-type headache, chronic sinusitis, ocular disorder, medication-overuse headache, psychosomatic) [37, 64]
- It is very important to know the warning features in childhood headache (see Box 2.1).

Table 2.6 Characteristic features of the common causes of both primary and secondary headaches from the history [37, 63, 93]

Type of headache	Characteristic features
Examples of primary headaches	
Migraine	– This is an acute recurrent headache; each attack lasts for <u>about 1–72 h</u>
	– It is characterized by a throbbing quality and a moderate-to-severe intensity
	– The headache is focal unilateral or bilateral or may switch from side to side
	– It is typically associated with anorexia, nausea, vomiting, pallor, light and sound sensitivity, and visual symptoms (such as flashing lights)
	– It is often triggered by stress, tiredness, or specific foods
	– It often occurs in the afternoon but sometimes awakens the child from sleep
	– It may be relieved by a short period of sleep
	– It is worsened by physical activity, so it disrupts the child's activities
	– Often there is a family history of migraines
	– It may occur with or without an aura (*Aura* is a neurologic alarm that a migraine will take place. It consists of visual, sensory, or language symptoms that develop over 5 min and last from 5 to 60 min. These symptoms are fully reversible)
	– **Note:** There are different types of migraines (e.g., migraine without aura, migraine with typical aura, vestibular migraine with vertigo, and chronic migraine). For each type of migraine, there are diagnostic criteria [94]

Table 2.6 (continued)

Type of headache	Characteristic features
Tension-type headaches (TTH)	– These tend to occur like a band around the head and can last for 5 min to 7 days – They are typically bilateral with a tightening quality – They occur late in the day or may last all day – They are mild-to-moderate in intensity and diffuse in location and are not affected by the activity – They do not interfere with sleep – They may be associated with anxiety, depression, or a stressful environment – There is an absence of other associated symptoms, like nausea, vomiting, or photophobia – They are relieved by stress reduction
Examples of secondary headaches	
Headache of increased intracranial pressure (ICP) (e.g., neoplasm, vascular malformation, or cystic structure)	– This is a chronic progressive headache of increasing severity or frequency – It frequently locates in the same position – It may have a throbbing, pressing, or sharp quality – It worsens by lying flat or coughing, and it is seldom relieved by any specific factor – It usually gets worse in the early morning and may awaken the child from sleep – It disrupts the child's activities – It may result in vomiting and may cause diplopia, due to a VI cranial nerve palsy
Headache of CNS infection (e.g., meningitis and infectious encephalitis)	– This is often of acute onset – It may be preceded by upper respiratory tract symptoms – It is associated with fever, neck or spine stiffness, focal neurologic signs, seizures, confusion, lethargy, arthralgia, myalgia, petechial or purpuric lesions, symptoms of raised ICP (e.g., vomiting, diplopia, ptosis, and apnea)
Intracranial hemorrhage	– This starts abruptly and develops rapidly – It presents as a very severe "thunderclap"; it is often described as "the worst pain in my life" – It may be associated with a loss of consciousness, nuchal rigidity, focal neurologic, in addition to deficits and seizures – The child may have a condition that may possibly lead to a hemorrhagic stroke, such as coagulopathy, hemoglobinopathy, or heart disease

History Station 2.23: Headache

- **Identity:** Age, sex
- **Chief complaint:** Headache
- **History of present illness:**
  1. Onset: Sudden or gradual
  2. Duration and time course of typical headache episode: A recent or chronic headache

Continued on the next page

3. Age of onset (if chronic)
4. Timing: Daytime or nighttime? What is the child doing when a typical headache begins?
5. Location: Temporal, suboccipital, retro-orbital, unilateral, bilateral, or switching from side to side
6. Character of pain: Band-like, throbbing, dull, sharp, thunderclap
7. Frequency of the headache and duration of each episode
8. Severity and progression: Does the headache cause the child to stop playing or interfere with normal activity? Does it wake the child from sleep? Does the headache become more frequent? Has it worsened or stayed the same?
9. Aura or prodrome: Blurred vision, visual scotomata, sensory disturbances, nausea, and/or vomiting
10. Aggravating or relieving factors: Exacerbation by sounds or light, exercising, straining, changing position, emotional upset, foods (e.g., cheese), or menses and relief by analgesics or sleep
11. Associated symptoms: Fever, nausea, vomiting, photophobia, diplopia, eye tearing, numbness, weakness, irritability, tiredness, agitation, loud crying, neck stiffness (suggests meningitis), vertigo, loss of consciousness
12. Triggers: Specific foods, activities, tiredness, stress, or events. Does the child have an idea about what triggers the headaches?
13. Has the headache preceded by upper respiratory tract symptoms?

- **Past history**: Past illnesses, depression, anxiety, motion sickness, head injuries, or allergies
- **Medication history**: Analgesics use (dosage and frequency of analgesics), ergotamine, triptan, vitamin A, or birth control pills, drug allergies
- **Development history:** Developmental delay, growth delay
- **Immunization history:** Influenza vaccine, hepatitis A vaccine
- **Family history:** Recurrent headaches or history of migraine in the family; parental description of their headaches; other neurologic, psychiatric, and general health conditions
- **Social history:** Stressful events, social withdrawal, school absences, emotional problems in school or at home, drug abuse, alcohol, cigarettes, travel, contact with animals
- **Review of systems:** Abdominal pain; diarrhea; gastrointestinal bleeding; pallor; skin rash; joint pain; changes in personality, intellectual skills, hearing, vision, memory, gait, balance, or strength; or postural lightheadedness

Key Points 2.23

- Acute recurrent throbbing headache suggests **a migraine**; headache that presents as a band around the head may suggest **a tension headache**; a thunderclap headache suggests **subarachnoid hemorrhage**.
- An acute-onset severe headache needs rapid assessment as it may require a specific and urgent treatment [64].
- A chronic progressive headache requires neuroimaging evaluation since it may suggest **an enlarging intracranial lesion**.

Box 2.1: Warning Features (Red Flags) in Childhood Headache [65]

- Recent headache onset
- First or worst headache
- Occipital location
- Increasing severity or frequency
- Headache causing awakening from sleep
- Neurologic abnormalities or visual changes
- Headache in the morning, associated with vomiting
- Persistent vomiting
- Behavioral changes

2.25 Seizure

- **A seizure** is a transient neurologic event resulting from abnormally excessive or synchronous neuronal activity in the brain [66].
- **An epilepsy** is the tendency to suffer from 2 or more unprovoked seizures.
- **A status epilepticus** is defined by Mikati and Hani as, "Continuous seizure activity or recurrent seizure activity without regaining of consciousness lasting for more than 5 minutes" [66].
- Seizures may be classified into [10, 66, 67]:
  - **Generalized seizures** (whole cortex is involved; consciousness is always impaired)
  - **Focal** (or **partial**) **seizures** (one area of cortex is involved; They may become generalized)
  - **Epilepsy syndromes**, which are symptomatic, idiopathic, or cryptogenic. For more details about the various types of seizures, see Table 2.7.
- A detailed history is indispensable in the initial assessment of a child with seizures (see History Station 2.24).

Table 2.7 Examples of various types of seizures, with a description of each one [66–68]

Type of seizure	Description/clinical features
Generalized tonic–clonic seizure	– The child falls to the ground unresponsive, with eye deviation or blinking – The initial generalized stiffness of limbs, body, and head (tonic phase) may be associated with cyanosis – The tonic phase is followed by arrhythmic jerking movements (clonic) – There may be salivary frothing and incontinence of urine or stool – There is a postictal period of decreased responsiveness or weakness
Tonic seizures	– These are breif seizures consisting of the sudden sustained contraction of extensor muscles – They are often associated with falls
Myoclonic seizures	– These are sudden, brief (usually <50 ms) involuntary contractions of muscles or muscle groups – The contractions can be singular or repetitive and are often irregular
Atonic seizures or drop attacks	– These are characterized by loss of postural tone and movement, typically lasting for a brief period (1–2 s) and associated with falls that may lead to facial injury
Absence seizures	– These occur in children aged between 4 and 12 years – They may be typical, atypical, or absence with special features – Typical absence seizures are generalized seizures consisting of an abrupt onset of unresponsiveness, loss of awareness, staring, and eye flutter – Often the only observed behaviors are lip smacking or semi-purposeful-appearing movements of the hands, with no falls – These are usually brief (2–15 s) and may occur hundreds of times per day – They may interfere with the child's activity and learning – They may be precipitated by hyperventilation for 3–5 min – There is no postictal drowsiness
Focal seizures	– Simple partial seizure: Consciousness is not impaired, with motor (can be tonic, clonic, myoclonic), sensory (visual, auditory, olfactory, gustatory, vertiginous, somatosensory), autonomic, or mixed symptoms – Complex partial seizure may be associated with impaired consciousness and automatisms – Partial seizures with secondarily generalized convulsions
Epileptic spasms (the preferred term over **infantile spasms**, because these can occur beyond infancy)	– These occur in infants aged between 3 months and 2 years – They consist of mixed flexion-extension, flexion, or, less commonly, extension of truncal and extremity muscles that is continued for 1–2 s and may associate with a cry – Attacks of epileptic spasm occur numerous times each day – They usually occur in clusters, either upon falling asleep or during early waking hours

Table 2.7 (continued)

Type of seizure	Description/clinical features
Febrile seizures	– These occur in children between the ages of 6 and 60 months and associate with fever (38 °C or higher) in the absence of CNS infection or any metabolic imbalance – Simple febrile seizures are primary generalized (usually tonic–clonic) and brief (last less than 15 min) and do not occur more than once within a day. The child with this type of seizure is neurologically and developmentally normal – Complex febrile seizures are focal, prolonged (last longer than 15 min), and/or repeated in the same illness (occur multiple times in 24 h)

History Station 2.24: Seizure

- **Identity:** Age
- **Chief complaint:** Abnormal body movement
- **History of present illness:**
  1. Antecedent: What happened in the hours before the spell? Was the child well or ill, feverish, excited or calm, tired or alert?
  2. Context: What happened immediately before the spell? What was the child doing? Were there any provoking factors?
  3. Onset: How did the spell start? Was there an aura (behavioral change, feeling of fear, a cry, epigastric discomfort or pain, irritability, lethargy)? Were there any warning signs, triggers for the spells (crying, boredom, anger, anxiety, trauma, or fever)? What was the first thing the child or witnesses noticed?
  4. Can the child tell when an episode will occur?
  5. Does the child remember the spells afterward? Can he/she describe what happens?
  6. Description of the event: Was the event witnessed? If so, what was noted during the attack? The color of the skin, lips, breathing changes, type of body movements: tonic–clonic movements, stiffness or floppiness, focal movement? What sort and where: limbs, face, mouth? Was saliva produced at the mouth? Eyes: What did the child's eyes do? Was the seizure associated with loss of consciousness, incontinence of urine or feces? Did the child experience a loss of responsiveness? Did the child speak or vocalize during the spell?
  7. How long did the event last (duration)? How did it resolve?
  8. Postictal phase: What did the child do after the attack? Postictal (weakness or paralysis, sleep, headache, confusion, injuries)? How long before getting back to normal?

Continued on the next page

- **Past history**:
  - **A**—Birth history: Maternal diabetes, complicated birth, prolonged labor with fetal distress, instrumental delivery, birth injury, and prolong resuscitation
  - **B**—Past medical and surgical history: Head trauma, meningitis, previous brain damage, metabolic disorders, illnesses, rheumatic fever, hospitalizations, history of febrile seizures, previous episodes of seizure. If there is epilepsy, ask about: When did it begin? What was the age of onset? What is the frequency of episodes? What were the results of electroencephalograms, CT scans, etc.?
- **Medication history:** Recent use of medications (e.g., antidepressants, stimulants, immunosuppressants, antibiotics, lithium, hypoglycemic agents, isoniazid), if the child on antiepileptic drugs (ask about type, dose, frequency of administration, recent modification of the dose, noncompliance with anticonvulsant medication), drug allergies
- **Development history:** Developmental delay, school performance
- **Immunization history:** Recent vaccination, e.g., MMR, diphtheria, tetanus, and acellular pertussis (DTaP)
- **Family history:** Family history of epilepsy or similar episodes, migraines, tremors, tics, streptococcal infection, rheumatic fever, sleep disturbance, Tourette syndrome, metabolic disorders, or liver disease
- **Social history:** Alcohol, drug addiction, lead exposure, impact of epilepsy on child's life
- **Review of Systems:** Diarrhea, vomiting, jaundice, pallor, weight loss, poor appetite, skin rash, hearing impairment, dyspnea, cyanosis, joint pain

Key Points 2.24

- Seizure in a neonate should always raise the concern for an underlying cause.
- Seizure in a febrile child aged <u>between 6 and 60 months</u> may suggest **febrile seizure** [66].
- A focal seizure may suggest **localized intracranial lesions**.
- Early onset of seizures, vomiting, and lethargy may suggest **a metabolic disorder**.
- Seizure associated with a recent headache, vomiting, lethargy, weakness, or alteration in gait may suggest **central nervous system (CNS) pathology,** or **space-occupying lesions** [68].

2.26 Lower-Limb Weakness

- **Weakness** can be defined as a decrement in the capability of the patient to move his/her muscles against resistance voluntarily and actively [69].
- **Paraplegia** refers to weakness of lower limbs due to dysfunction of the nervous system at the level of the peripheral nerves, spinal cord, or brain [70].
- Paraplegia can be classified as either congenital or acquired.
- Acquired paraplegias can be divided according to the timing of onset into:
  - **Acute paraplegias** evolving over a period from minutes to hours, for example, spinal cord infarction or trauma
  - **Subacute paraplegias** evolving over a period from hours to days, e.g., poliomyelitis, Guillain–Barré syndrome, or transverse myelitis
  - **Chronic paraplegias** evolving over a period from weeks to months, e.g., tumors
- A thorough history is essential to reach a precise diagnosis in a child with lower-limb weakness (see History Station 2.25 and Table 2.8).

Table 2.8 Short case scenarios of the most important causes of lower-limb weakness in children [26, 67, 69, 70]

Short case scenarios	Diagnosis and special point(s) in favor
A 6-year-old child presents with symmetric and ascending lower-limb weakness, which started gradually and progressed over 3 days. The condition began as a transient numbness in lower limbs and paresthesia, followed by weakness, which is accompanied by buttock and leg pain. The mother stated that the child was suffering from a respiratory tract infection 10 days ago	**Guillain–Barré syndrome (GBS)** – Guillain–Barré syndrome is uncommon in children aged less than 3 years – It starts and progresses over a period ranging from hours to days – The paralysis is progressive, symmetric, and ascending; proximal and distal muscles are involved relatively symmetrically, but asymmetry is found in 9% of patients – Weakness usually starts in the lower limbs and gradually involves the trunk, the upper extremities, and, eventually, the bulbar muscles – Sensory symptoms are common – Autonomic nerve involvement can cause arrhythmia or bowel and bladder dysfunction – In about 50% of patients with GBS, the paralysis follows a gastrointestinal or respiratory infection by about 10 days – Weakness usually reaches its maximal severity by 1 month after onset

(continued)

Table 2.8 (continued)

Short case scenarios	Diagnosis and special point(s) in favor
A 3-year-old male child presents, after an intramuscular injection, with weakness of his left leg, starting gradually and evolving within 2 days to involve the left-upper hands and accompanied by a low-grade fever, malaise, muscle pain, and severe headache, as well as nuchal rigidity	**Poliomyelitis** – Flaccid paralysis or paresis is usually asymmetric and commonly involves one leg, and then one upper limb is involved. The proximal areas of the limbs are more affected than the distal areas – Bulbar weakness may occur – The paralysis may be preceded by a history of an intramuscular injection in half of the patients – Bowel and bladder dysfunction may occur; it often accompanies paralysis of the lower extremities – Sensory symptoms are not present in a child with poliomyelitis; their presence should raise the concern for a disease other than poliomyelitis
A 9-year-old male child presents at the emergency room with acute symmetric weakness of the lower extremities, associated with anesthesia and reduced sensory perception below the level of the umbilicus. The weakness was preceded by thoracic back pain and bilateral lower-limb numbness. According to the mother, the child has no history of trauma	**Transverse myelitis** – Rapid progression of weakness over a period lasting from a few hours to a few days – The patient may present with thoracic back pain, lower-limb numbness, and then acute uniform symmetric (or asymmetric) weakness of the lower extremities, associated with anesthesia and reduced sensory perception below the level of the lesion – Progressive bladder or bowel dysfunction – May be preceded by viral infection, bacterial infection, or vaccination
An adolescent male presents with progressive lower-limb weakness associated with a high-grade fever, headache, vomiting, neck stiffness, limb pain, and severe localized back pain, which increased in severity with cough or flexion	**Epidural abscess** – Limb pain starts 3–6 days after the onset of back pain, followed by a progressive limb weakness and bladder dysfunction
A school-aged child presents with acute right lower-limb weakness occurring within a few hours after trauma to the back and associated with an inability to pass urine	**Traumatic paralysis** – Acute asymmetric limb weakness occurs from a few hours to a few days after the trauma – This is typically associated with bowel and bladder dysfunction
An adolescent female presents with lower-limb weakness that evolved over 6 weeks and associated with headache, vomiting, and behavioral changes. She is a known case of a brain tumor	**Brain tumor** – The patient usually has a history of known brain tumor or a history of a lower-limb weakness – A severe headache may occur when there is a hemorrhage inside the tumor

Table 2.8 (continued)

Short case scenarios	Diagnosis and special point(s) in favor
An adolescent male presents with gait difficulty and lower-limb weakness that evolved over 3 months and associated with back pain and loss of sensation over the affected limb	**Spinal cord tumor** – This usually presents with a slowly progressive lower-limb weakness, accompanied by sensory loss and back pain – It may be accompanied by bowel and bladder dysfunction

---

History Station 2.25: Lower-Limb Weakness

- **Identity:** Age, sex, address, nationality
- **Chief complaint:** Lower-limb weakness
- **History of present illness:**
    1. Timing of weakness onset: Acute, subacute, or chronic
    2. Duration/specific date of onset
    3. Progression: Increasing, static, or improving
    4. Site: Where did it start? Is it proximal or distal involvement? Is it symmetrical or asymmetrical?
    5. Evolution: Are both limbs affected simultaneously or one after the other?
    6. Degree of weakness: Ability of the child to walk, to lift arm to comb hair, to lift an object, or to move leg in bed (if unable to walk)
    7. Associated symptoms: Fever, headaches, neck or back pain, disturbed level of consciousness, seizure, involuntary movements, tremors, dysphagia, mouth deviation, aphonia, hoarseness
    8. Sensory loss, tingling, or any changes in sensation? If so, in what distribution?
    9. Bowel and bladder dysfunction
    10. Cranial nerve involvement: Visual problems, hearing and speech problems, drooling of saliva
    11. Precipitating factors: Fever, convulsion, exercise, trauma, intramuscular injections, or snake bite
    12. Preceded by gastroenteritis, flu-like illness (especially in the last 10 days)
    13. Recovery: Rapid recovery, slow regression over a period of time, or persisting indefinitely
- **Past history**:
    A—Birth history: Preterm, breech presentation, prolonged labor, delayed cry at birth, birth asphyxia
    B—Past medical and surgical history: Previous limb weakness, numbness, or other neurologic symptoms, head trauma, epilepsy, tuberculosis, dia-

Continued on the next page

betes mellitus, hypertension, autoimmune disorders, or multiple sclerosis
- **Medication history:** Recent use of medications (e.g., steroids), drug allergies
- **Immunization history:** Recent vaccination, poliomyelitis vaccine (injectable or oral), rabies vaccine, influenza vaccine, meningococcal conjugate vaccine, and tetanus toxoid
- **Feeding/dietary history:** Type of feeding, ingestion of home-canned foods, undercooked meat
- **Family history:** Family history of leg weakness, muscular dystrophies, neuropathies, myopathies, myasthenia gravis, hypertension, diabetes mellitus, epilepsy, or migraine
- **Social history:** Poor sanitation, crowding, water contamination, educational achievements, exposure to toxins (organophosphorus, inorganic lead, arsenic)
- **Review of systems:** Dark urine (rhabdomyolysis), dyspnea, diarrhea, vomiting, myalgia, recent weight loss (brain tumor, tuberculosis)

Key Points 2.25

- Weakness that occurs and deteriorates suddenly without trauma may suggest **subarachnoid hemorrhage, stroke,** or **brain neoplasm with hemorrhage** [69].
- Weakness that occurs in conjunction with headache, particularly in children with focal neurological signs or progressive morning vomiting, should raise the concern for **an intracranial mass lesion** [69].
- Subacute, chronic, or indolent presentations of weakness should raise the possibility of **neuropathies** (e.g., Guillain–Barré syndrome) or **myopathies** (e.g., muscular dystrophy).
- The occurrence of weakness in combination with a seizure may point to **acute intracranial hemorrhage** or **stroke**. It may also result from a self-limited **Todd paralysis** [69].
- Weakness that is preceded by a history of viral infection, bacterial infection (particularly *Campylobacter jejuni* infection), surgery, or vaccination is suggestive of **Guillain–Barré syndrome**, the most common cause of acute flaccid paralysis in children [26].

2.27 Coma and Confusion

• **Coma** is an alteration of consciousness with loss of both wakefulness and awareness. The comatose patient appears to be asleep and unresponsive and cannot be aroused. It is a transient state, whereby the patient regains his/her consciousness or progresses to the minimally conscious state, persistent vegetative state, or may progress to brain death [71, 72].

History Station 2.26: Coma and Confusion

• **Identity:** Age, sex
• **Chief complaint(s):** Loss of consciousness, disturbed level of consciousness
• **History of present illness:**
  1. Onset: Sudden or gradual
  2. Timing of symptom onset and duration
  3. Activity and symptoms prior to onset; recent fever, bacterial or viral illnesses. What happened immediately before the event? Was there history of head trauma? If so, find out the time between trauma and loss of consciousness.
  4. Progression of the condition
  5. Associated symptoms: Fever, neck pain, convulsion, double vision, headache
  6. Recent weight changes or other constitutional abnormalities (may suggest **endocrine dysfunction** or **an oncologic process**)
  7. Recent nausea, vomiting, or headache (may suggest raised ICP)
• **Past history:**
  A—Birth history: In the case of a newborn <1 week old, consider the history of birth asphyxia, birth injury to the brain
  B—Past medical and surgical history: Prior episodes of unexplained coma, diabetes, heart disease, inborn errors of metabolism, immunosuppression, brain tumor, seizure disorder, depression, suicide attempts, surgery
• **Medication history:** Toxin ingestion or drug overdose: What medications are in the home? (Insulin, oral antidiabetics, narcotics, anticholinergics, sedatives, salicylate, psychotropics, lithium, etc.), drug allergies
• **Developmental history**: Developmental delay
• **Immunization history:** Recent vaccination
• **Family history:** Family history of the same condition, heart disease, metabolic disease
• **Social history:** Travel, recent sick contact, child abuse, psychological stress, alcohol or drug abuse
• **Review of systems:** Nausea, vomiting, diarrhea, jaundice, polyuria, polydipsia, pallor, peripheral or facial edema, skin rash

Key Points 2.26

- Mental status deterioration that starts gradually is suggestive of **an infectious process, slowly expanding intracranial mass lesion,** or **metabolic abnormality** [71, 72].
- Coma that is preceded by headache with positional changes or with Valsalva maneuver may suggest raised **ICP from hydrocephalus** or **intracranial mass lesion**.
- **Coma** associated with headache and neck pain or stiffness may suggest **meningeal irritation** due to inflammation, infection, or intracranial hemorrhage.
- **Fever in a comatose child** suggests **infection**. However, the absence of fever does not rule out infection, especially in children under 6 months of age or those who are immunocompromised [71].
- Mental status fluctuation or abnormal movements may suggest **postictal state** or **non-convulsive seizures**.
- A previous history of unexplained episodes of coma may suggest **recurrent toxic ingestions, intermittent metabolic disease,** or **Munchausen by proxy syndrome**.
- Pre-existing neurological abnormalities and developmental delay are suggestive of **inborn errors of metabolism** or **a prolonged postictal state**.
- Coma in a child with a known cardiac disease should raise the possibility of **circulatory collapse** or **hypoxic-ischemic encephalopathy**.

2.28   Skin Rash

- **Rash** is a general term referring to any skin eruption.
- Although a comprehensive physical examination is essential to assess the condition of the child with a skin eruption, a thorough history and precise description of the eruption can be very helpful in removing any obstacle to accurate diagnosis (see History Station 2.27 and Table 2.9).

Table 2.9 Short cases history of some diseases that may cause a skin rash [13, 73, 74, 90]

Short case history	Diagnosis and special points in favor
A 10-month-old female infant presents with an erythematous maculopapular rash that started at the scalp, hairline, and face and then moved caudally to involve the whole body. The child also has high fever, dry cough, runny nose, and red eyes that started 2 days prior to the onset of the rash. She had not received any vaccinations	**Measles (rubeola)** – This presents as high fever, dry cough, coryza, runny nose, conjunctivitis, and malaise – Koplik spots (bluish-white sand-like papules on a red base on the buccal surfaces may present on day 1–2 of fever, over buccal mucosa) and skin rash – The rash is initially erythematous and maculopapular but then becomes confluent

Table 2.9   (continued)

Short case history	Diagnosis and special points in favor
A 7-year-old male child presents an erythematous maculopapular rash, preceded by 2 days of fever and pharyngitis. The rash appeared initially on the neck and upper trunk and spread rapidly to cover the whole body. It was accentuated in the axillae and antecubital, inguinal, and popliteal creases, while the palms and soles were spared	**Scarlet fever** – This starts with fever and pharyngitis, followed by the rash in 1–2 days – A fine erythematous maculopapular rash with a sandpaper texture appears initially on the neck and upper trunk and then spreads rapidly to cover the entire body – The patient presents with flushed face and circumoral pallor – Initially, the tongue is white, coated, and furred (white strawberry tongue); then, within 4–5 days, it becomes red and swollen (red strawberry tongue) – Within several days, the rash fades with a skin peeling
A 4-year-old female child presents with a pinkish maculopapular rash, which began on the face and then spread to cover the entire body. The rash was preceded by an upper-respiratory tract prodrome and associated with painful eye movements. According to the mother, postauricular small nodules were also noticed	**Rubella** – Rubella may start with an upper-respiratory tract prodrome, followed by the rash – The rash is a fine, pinkish maculopapular rash that begins on the face and spreads to involve the whole body. It typically lasts about 3 days – It may be associated with painful eye movements, which are characteristic – Lymphadenopathy is prominent, especially in the suboccipital and postauricular nodes
A 3-year-old male child presents with a bright-red rash over his cheeks, with pallor around the mouth. The rash spread rapidly on the trunk, buttocks, and the extensor surface of extremities. It was associated with a low-grade fever, headache, and mild upper respiratory symptoms that started before the onset of the rash	**Erythema infectiosum** – A reticulate rash spreads rapidly on the trunk, buttocks, and extensor surface of extremities – Red papules that coalesce on the face may appear as "slapped cheeks" – The palms and soles may be involved
A 10-month-old infant presents with a rose-colored skin rash, preceded by upper-respiratory symptoms and a high fever (>40°). The rash started on the trunk and spread to the face, neck, and limbs. It coincided with the abrupt remission of the fever	**Roseola infantum** – Roseola usually occurs in children younger than 4 years old (typical age 9–12 months) – The rash consists of rose-colored discrete blanching, small, raised lesions start on the trunk and spread to the face, neck, and limbs. It may last 1–3 days – The rash coincided with the abrupt remission of the fever – A febrile seizure may occur

(continued)

Table 2.9 (continued)

Short case history	Diagnosis and special points in favor
A 5-year-old male child presents with a skin rash, preceded by 2 days of fever, malaise, and poor appetite. The rash started as erythematous macules and papules but rapidly developed into small vesicles. These lesions existed simultaneously in varying phases of development on the face, trunk, and scalp, with minimal involvement of the distal extremities. The mucous membranes were involved, and the palms and soles were spared	**Chickenpox (varicella)** – Chickenpox may be preceded by fever, malaise, poor appetite, headache, and abdominal pain – The rash progresses from erythematous macules to papules, to fluid-filled vesicles, and occurs in the dermatome (or in two adjacent dermatomes) and finally crusts
A 2-year-old male child presents with a high-grade fever not relieved by paracetamol, lasted for a 6-day duration, associated with irritability, and a morbilliform rash started in the groin region. The child also has red eyes, cracked red lips, and cervical lymphadenopathy	**Kawasaki disease** – Kawasaki disease usually occurs in children between 6 months and 5 years of age. (the median age is 2–3 years old.) It is rare in children <3 months of age – The rash of Kawasaki disease may be morbilliform, scarlatiniform, pustular, urticarial, or erythema multiforme-like – The oropharyngeal changes are bright-red and fissured lips with some crusting, oral erythema, and a strawberry tongue – Bilateral non-purulent conjunctivitis occurs in >90% of patients – Edema and erythema of the palms and soles may occur, and peeling of fingers and toes occurs in the second or third week
An 8-month-old unwell male infant presented with an 11-h history of fever, lethargy, and a spreading purpuric rash over the trunk, extremities, and palate. The symptoms were preceded by mild upper-respiratory symptoms	**Meningococcemia** – Meningococcemia presents as a set of mild upper-respiratory symptoms, followed by fever, malaise, headache, and skin rash, which may appear as a non-blanching maculopapular purpuric rash and petechiae and then ecchymosis over the trunk, limbs, and palate
A 7-year-old female presents with intensely itchy wheals with surrounding erythema over her chest, back, and abdomen. The lesions lasted for less than 12 h, to be replaced by new lesions at other sites. There were no other associated symptoms	**Urticaria** – Urticaria typically presents as a pruritic raised central wheal with surrounding erythema – Lesions usually last for a few hours (less than 24 h)
A 6-month-old male child presents with a 2-month history of recurrent pruritic erythematous, exudative, crusty, and oozy lesions, distributed over the cheeks, scalp, trunk, and extensor aspects of the extremities. He had a family history of asthma	**Atopic dermatitis** – This presents with a chronic and recurrent pruritic rash that varies with the child's age – Infantile (from 2 months to 2 years) (described in this case) – In older children (from 2 years to adolescence): lichenified, dry, itchy plaques involving flexural aspects (neck, antecubital, popliteal)

History Station 2.27: Skin Rash

- **Identity:** Age, sex, address, ethnicity/race
- **Chief complaint:** Rash
- **History of present illness:**
  1. Onset: Acute vs. gradual
  2. Duration: When did the rash appear?
  3. Site of the first appearance of the rash: Where did the rash first appear? What did it look like when it first appeared?
  4. Features of the rash:
     - Location, pattern of spread (e.g., trunk to extremities)
     - Configuration of the rash: What did it resemble?
     - Color of the rash
     - Progression of the rash over time, changes in appearance, or distribution over time
  5. Associated symptoms: Fever (if there is fever, ask about timing of onset of the rash in relation to fever), pruritus, scaling, joint pain, neck pain or stiffness, and abdominal pain. If the child has any symptoms accompanying the rash, then ask, "Did these symptoms start before, with, or after the onset of the rash?" How long has the child had these symptoms?
  6. Factors that worsen or precipitate the rash: Exposure to irritants, allergens, insect bites, trauma at the site of the rash, change in seasons, cold, or sun exposure
- **Past history:**
  A—Birth history: Maternal infections, advance maternal age, prematurity, low birth weight, twinning
  B—Past medical and surgical history: Prior history of skin rashes (e.g., chickenpox, measles, etc.), allergic rhinitis, asthma, urticaria, eczema, IBD, SLE, renal disease, neurological disease, malnutrition, immunodeficiency, diabetes, hospitalizations, or surgery
- **Medication history:** Treatments that have been tried, exposure to certain medications (e.g., antibiotics, antiepileptics, steroids, chemotherapy, etc.), topical therapies may be relevant to the child's condition (e.g., neomycin, diphenhydramine, and certain anesthetics, if applied topically, these may cause contact dermatitis), drug allergies
- **Immunization history:** Recent vaccination, vaccination status, MMR vaccine (measles, mumps, rubella)
- **Family history:** Does anyone else in the family have a similar rash? Is there a family history of atopic disease? Allergic rhinitis? Asthma? SLE? IBD?
- **Social history:** Exposure to persons with rash, travel and outdoor activities, alcohol, substance abuse, home situation, psychologic stress, sexual activity (secondary syphilis and disseminated gonococcal infection, molluscum contagiosum, or scabies). Are there pregnant contacts?
- **Review of systems:** Malaise, headache, decreased activity, conjunctivitis, coryza, cough, sore throat, wheezing, rhinorrhea, decreased appetite, weight loss, diarrhea, photosensitivity, etc.

Key Points 2.27

- The configuration of the rash may be very helpful. The rash of herpes zoster is characterized by a dermatomal configuration; allergic contact dermatitis may present in a linear or geometric configuration, while linear IgA disease (LAD) of childhood is typically characterized by annular configuration of bullae and vesicles [73].
- A generalized erythematous macular rash associated with fever, cough, and nasal congestion is suggestive of **a viral exanthem**.
- In an ill-appearing child, the presence of petechiae and purpura associated with fever should raise the concern for **a serious bacterial infection**, such as meningococcemia.
- A pruritic rash may suggest **atopic dermatitis**, **contact dermatitis**, **urticaria**, **chickenpox**, **scabies**, **diabetes**, or **HIV/AIDS** [74].

2.29   Fever

- **Fever** can be defined as a rectal temperature ≥38.0 °C [75–77].
- A rectal temperature of more than 40 °C is called "hyperpyrexia" [75].
- Body temperature tends to be lower in the early morning and peaks in the evening, with a normal range of 36.6–37.9 °C (taken rectally) [75, 77].
- **Fever of unknown origin (FUO)** can be defined as a daily rectal temperature >38.3 °C that is present for more than 14 days with no apparent source, in spite of taking a complete history, conducting a thorough physical examination, and carrying out preliminary laboratory studies [78].
- In the pediatric population, the most common cause of fever is a viral infection [77].

History Station 2.28: Fever

- **Identity:** Age, sex, address, ethnicity/race
- **Chief complaint:** Fever
- **History of present illness:**
  1. Time of onset and duration
  2. Degree of fever: How high has the temperature been? How was it measured (orally, axillary, rectally, or tympanically)?
  3. Pattern of fever
  4. Has the child's activity level changed? Is he/she more sleepy than usual or irritable?
  5. Associated symptoms: Shivering, rigors, chills, cough, sputum, rhinorrhea, sore throat, headache, red eyes, or skin rash

Continued on the next page

6. Are there symptoms of a specific illness?
7. Were there recent tick bites?
- **Past history**:
  A—Birth history: Maternal infections, premature rupture of membranes, meconium-stained amniotic fluid, low Apgar score at birth, prematurity, and low birth weight (these may be risk factors for neonatal sepsis).
  B—Past medical and surgical history: Hospitalized for an infectious illness, medical illnesses, (asthma, diabetes, sickle-cell anemia, congenital heart disease, immunodeficiency, etc.), recent dental procedure, surgery
- **Medication history:** Recent use of medications, e.g., cimetidine, steroids, anticholinergic agents, antibiotics (penicillins, cephalosporins, sulfonamides, etc.), acetaminophen, anticonvulsants, and methylphenidate (may cause medication-related fever), drug allergies
- **Immunization history:** Recent vaccination—what immunizations has the child received?
- **Feeding/dietary history:** Consumption of unpasteurized milk (brucellosis), poor feeding, ingestion of raw meat or fish, pica or dirt ingestion (*Toxoplasma gondii* infection)
- **Family history:** Another family members with fever, familial Mediterranean fever, connective-tissue disease
- **Social history:** Exposure to animals, recent travel, past residence, alcohol, smoking, ill contacts, well-water ingestion (giardiasis), exposure to tuberculosis or hepatitis
- **Review of systems:** Change in mental status, change in behavior or activity (suggests brain tumor, tuberculosis), lethargy, irritability, seizure, neck stiffness, abdominal pain, dysuria, frequency, new onset of incontinence, ear pain, vomiting, night sweats, diarrhea, decreased appetite, weight loss, difficulty in swallowing, bone or joint pain, vaginal discharge, etc.

Key Points 2.28

- Well-appearing infants (<2 months of age) with a fever ($\geq$38.0 ° C) but without an identifiable source of infection are at risk for **occult serious bacterial infections**. It is uncommon for them to have the common viral infections of older infants and children because of passive immunity from their mothers [76].
- The pattern of fever may point to the underlying etiology: **Continuous** (e.g., typhoid fever), **remittent** (as in most viral or bacterial diseases), **intermittent** (e.g., malaria, endocarditis), **hectic** (e.g., Kawasaki disease), **quotidian** (e.g., malaria caused by *P. vivax*), **double quotidian** (e.g., kala-azar), **periodic** (e.g., brucellosis), or **recurrent fever** (e.g., familial Mediterranean fever, which is common in certain ethnic groups, such as Arab, Armenian, and Turkish) [77].

2.30 Pallor

- The term **pallor** refers to the perception of a decreased redness in the skin and mucous membranes, commonly occurring due to a decrement in the circulating hemoglobin level (e.g., anemia) or poor peripheral perfusion (e.g., shock) [79, 80].
- Pallor may be caused by **hematologic** or **non-hematologic** etiologies [79].

History Station 2.29: Pallor

- **Identity:** Age, sex, address and birthplace, ethnicity/race
- **Chief complaint:** Pallor
- **History of present illness:**
  1. Onset: Sudden onset (suggests hemolysis); gradual onset (suggests iron-deficiency anemia)
  2. Duration of pallor
  3. Associated symptoms: Jaundice (suggests hemolysis); systemic symptoms (e.g., fever, fatigue, growth failure, weight loss, or lymphadenopathy), which may suggest malignancy; and symptoms of cardiovascular compromise (e.g., easy fatigability; dyspnea, at rest or with exercise; orthopnea; chest pain; palpitation)
  4. Is there a blood loss from anywhere (melena, bleeding per rectum, hematuria, or menorrhagia)?
  5. History of seizures, syncope, or recent trauma
  6. Has the child had a recent infection? (That is the most common cause of mild anemia in children.)
- **Past history:**
  A—Birth history: A complete prenatal history, prematurity (increased risk of iron deficiency), neonatal jaundice
  B—Past medical and surgical history: Hemoglobinopathy, G6PD deficiency, history of chronic illnesses, chronic renal disease, hypothyroidism, juvenile idiopathic arthritis, blood transfusion, gallstones, abnormal bleeding, recent surgery, splenectomy, cholecystectomy
- **Medication history:** Recent use of medications, e.g., methotrexate (can induce a megaloblastic anemia); chloramphenicol, sulfa drugs, anticonvulsants, and cancer chemotherapeutic agents (may cause aplastic anemia); oxidants, such as sulfonamide or nitrofurantoin (may induce hemolytic anemias)
- **Feeding/dietary history:** Consumption of cow's milk before 12 months of age and high cow's milk intake (greater than 24 ounces per day) are associated with iron deficiency. Dietary habits, meat ingestion, vegetarian diets, pica (associated with iron-deficiency anemia)

Continued on the next page

- **Family history:** Consanguinity, hemolytic anemia (e.g., hemoglobinopathies, G6PD deficiency, and spherocytosis), splenectomy, gallstones, early cholecystectomy (may suggest a previously undiagnosed hemolytic anemia), jaundice. Are the child's parents pale without a history of anemia?
- **Social history:** Living conditions, poverty, recent exposure to toxins
- **Review of systems:** Bone or joint pain, abdominal pain, diarrhea, skin rash, headache, mental status changes

Key Points 2.29

- Acute onset of pallor may suggest **hemolytic anemia**, especially if associated with jaundice and dark-colored urine, while a gradually developed pallor may imply **iron-deficiency anemia** or **bone-marrow aplasia** [80].
- Exposure to drugs or toxins may cause anemia from hemolysis or bone-marrow suppression.
- Iron deficiency anemia is a common cause of pallor in toddlers and adolescents, especially girls [81].
- **Acute or chronic blood loss** and **hemolytic disease of the newborn (HDN)** are common causes of anemia in neonates [79].
- Pallor in children <6 months of age may suggest **a congenital anemia** or **isoimmunization** [82].
- Consumption of large quantities of cow's milk may suggest **iron-deficiency anemia** [80].
- A sudden onset of pallor with lethargy should raise the possibility of **an acute process**, such as **acute anemia**, **hypoglycemia**, or **a fulminant bacterial infection**.
- **G6PD deficiency** and **thalassemia** are common in children of Mediterranean or Asian descent [79].
- Pallor of the child's parents without a history of anemia may suggest **a constitutional pallor**.
- A slow onset of pallor with other major systemic symptoms suggests **anemia of chronic diseases**, such as **cystic fibrosis**, **nephrotic syndrome**, or **malignancy** [79, 80].

2.31   Bleeding and Bruising

- **Excessive bleeding** and **bruises** result from disruptions in one or more of the three phases of normal hemostasis: constriction of blood vessels (**vascular phase**), formation of the platelet plug (**primary hemostasis**), and formation of the fibrin thrombus (**secondary hemostasis**) [83].

- Bleeding disorders can be **inherited**, e.g., von Willebrand disease and hemophilia, or **acquired**, e.g., vitamin K deficiency, disseminated intravascular coagulation (DIC), liver or renal diseases, post-surgery, infection, medications, massive transfusion, malignancy, and autoimmunity or alloimmunity [84].

History Station 2.30: Bleeding and Bruising

- **Identity:** Age, sex, ethnicity/race
- **Chief complaint(s): Bleeding**: gum bleeding, epistaxis, hematemesis, melena, hematuria, joint pain and swelling (bleeding into joints), or menorrhagia (menstrual flow >7 days), or **bruising**
- **History of present illness:**
  1. Time of onset and duration of bleeding and bruising: Is the symptom acute or chronic?
  2. Site of bleeding or bruising
  3. Amount of blood loss and size of bruising
  4. Associated symptoms: Fever, pallor, jaundice, bleeding from other sites
  5. Precipitating factors: A history of recent trauma, a history of rat poison ingestion (suggests warfarin toxicity)
  6. Frequency of bleeding: Is it recurrent? How often do the bleeding events occur?
  7. A history of a viral prodrome or recent illness
  8. Concurrent disease and the overall health of the child
- **Past history**:
  A—Birth history: Any maternal disease, including maternal ITP, maternal drug use (is the mother taking phenytoin?) (suggests vitamin K deficiency), delayed wound healing or bleeding from the umbilical stump after birth (suggests factor XIII deficiency)
  B—Past medical and surgical history: Has the child had bleeding or bruise previously? If so, how often? How was it controlled? (If epistaxis, ask about history of packing and cauterization.) Prolonged bleeding after minor trauma, after loss of primary teeth, or after minor surgery (e.g., circumcision), repeated hemarthroses, blood or platelet transfusions in the past or recently, bleeding at injection sites, recurring infections, recent surgery, obstetric and gynecologic problems (if adolescent female, take full menstrual history).
- **Medication history:** Anticoagulants (e.g., heparin and warfarin); antiplatelet drugs (e.g., aspirin, ibuprofen, diclofenac, etc.); antihistamines; steroids; quinidine; digoxin; antiepileptic drugs (e.g., valproic acid, can cause immune-mediated thrombocytopenia); penicillins and cephalosporins (can also cause platelet dysfunction, particularly in children with a systemic disease); oral contraceptives; drug allergies
- **Immunization history:** Has the patient developed large hematomas at vaccination sites?

Continued on the next page

- **Feeding/dietary history:** Type of feeding, exclusive breastfeeding (consider vitamin K deficiency)
- **Family history:** Consanguinity, bleeding disorders in the family, prolonged bleeding after minor surgery, obsretric and gynecologic history of female relatives
- **Social history:** Family stress, history of child abuse, availability of rodenticides in the home
- **Review of systems:** Bone or joint pain, abdominal pain, weight loss, neurologic manifestations (seen in meningococcemia or thrombotic thrombocytopenic purpura)

Key Points 2.30

- Bleeding and bruising 2–7 days after birth may suggest **a hemorrhagic disease of the newborn** [83, 84].
- **Purpuric lesions** indicate disruptions in the **vascular phase** or **primary hemostasis**.
- **Hemarthroses** and **deep bleeding** may point to disorders of **secondary hemostasis**.
- Acute onset of purpura suggests **an acquired disorder**.
- A history of recurrent purpura since infancy is suggestive of **an inherited disorder**.
- A history of a viral prodrome suggests **hemolytic–uremic syndrome (HUS), idiopathic thrombocytopenic purpura (ITP)**, or **Henoch–Schönlein Purpura (HSP)**.
- An abrupt onset of bruising or bleeding in a healthy child aged under 10 years is suggestive of **ITP** [83].
- Acute bleeding from multiple sites in an unhealthy child may suggest **DIC** [84].
- A palpable purpura on the extensor surfaces of the arms, legs, and buttocks, associated with abdominal pain, hematuria, joint pain, or arthritis in a 3- to 10-year-old child should raise the concern for **HSP**, especially if preceded by a viral prodrome [83].

2.32   Joint Pain

- **Joint pain** can be inflammatory, mechanical, or idiopathic [85].
- **Inflammatory joint pain (arthritis)** is often persistent and worse after a period of inactivity or in the morning with morning stiffness; it is generally relieved by exercise.
- **Mechanical joint pain** is frequently intermittent, exacerbated by activity, and relieved by rest, usually preceded by a history of trauma.

- **Idiopathic joint pain** is most severe and unremitting, usually occurring in conjunction with fatigue and poor sleep. It is usually associated with significant functional impairment, though there is no recognizable organic pathology [85, 86].
- In addition, **joint pain** may also be caused by osteomyelitis, tumors, metabolic abnormalities (e.g., rickets, hypo-/hyperthyroidism, diabetes), or genetic disorders. For more details, see Table 2.10.
- **Arthritis** is a term used when there is a limitation of movement in a joint associated with evidence of inflammation in the joint (i.e., swelling, warmth, redness, tenderness, along with pain with movement) [87].
- **Arthralgia** can be defined as joint pain without evidence of inflammation in the joint space. The pain or discomfort originates in the joint itself [87].

Table 2.10 Short case scenarios of different causes of joint pain in children [26, 85–89]

Short case scenarios	Diagnosis and special points in favor
A 10-year-old child presents with a 3-day history of right-knee pain. It is intermittent, exacerbated by exercise, and relieved by rest. There was a history of trauma to the joint	**Traumatic joint pain** – This is more common in older children and adolescents – It is frequently intermittent, exacerbated by exercise, and relieved by rest – It is preceded by a history of trauma
An adolescent male patient presents with a 5-week history of right ankle joint pain and swelling, associated with lower back pain, malaise, red eyes, and dysuria. Further review of symptoms showed that he had diarrhea 3 weeks ago	**Reactive arthritis** (Reiter syndrome) – This is characterized by a transient joint swelling (<6 weeks), often of the ankles or knees – It may follow (or rarely accompany) extra-articular infection – Although the enteric bacteria are the common cause in children, viral infections and sexually transmitted infections are also involved in adolescents
A 7-year-old boy presents with a 2-week history of migratory joint pain and swelling, affecting several large joints in a quick succession. Each joint was affected for a few days. The child also has fever and chest pain. According to the mother, there was a history of pharyngitis 3 weeks prior to the onset of symptoms	**Acute rheumatic fever** – It is most common in children between 5 and 15 years of age – Migratory arthritis affects several large joints in a quick succession. – Each joint is affected for less than 1 week, while the entire polyarthritis infrequently continues for more than 4 weeks – It occurs after group A streptococcus pharyngitis by about 2–3 weeks
A 5-year-old male child presents with a rapid onset of joint pain, associated with swelling, warmth, redness, fever, and restricted joint movement. The pain is exacerbated by any range of motion	**Septic arthritis** – This is a rapid onset of joint pain associated with fever – It involves joint swelling, warmth, redness, and restricted joint movement – Joint pain is exacerbated by any range of motion

Table 2.10 (continued)

Short case scenarios	Diagnosis and special points in favor
A 5-year-old male child presents with a limp and hip pain, preceded by upper respiratory infection. The child is able to move his hip through some range of motion without pain	**Transient synovitis of the hip** – This is most common in male children aged 3–9 years – It may be preceded by or occur concurrently with an upper respiratory infection – It commonly affects the hip joint, causing a limp, along with hip, thigh, or knee pain – The child appears nontoxic and able to move his hip through some range of motion without pain, in contrast to septic arthritis and osteomyelitis
A 12-year-old male presents with a history of pain and swelling in his left knee and ankle for more than 6 weeks. The pain is worsened in the morning and improves throughout the day with activity	**Juvenile idiopathic arthritis** – This occurs in children under 16 years and lasts for more than 6 weeks – The pain is worsened in the morning and improves throughout the day with activity – It has different subtypes: oligoarthritis (60%), polyarthritis (24%), enthesitis-related (7%), and systemic (Still's disease) (9%)
An adolescent female presents with pain and swelling of her right ankle and interphalangeal joints of the index finger of the left hand, along with associated photosensitive facial rash, mainly over the nose and cheeks. In the last 3 days, she also developed a mouth ulcer	**Systemic lupus erythematosus (SLE)** – This is more common in adolescent females – Arthritis is often asymmetric polyarthritis, involving both large and small joints – It is associated with other symptoms of SLE, such as the typical skin rash
A 4-year-old male child presents with knee pain, associated with a colicky abdominal pain and purpuric rash on the buttocks and thighs. According to the mother, the child had a history of an upper-respiratory tract infection 2 weeks prior to the onset of symptoms	**Henoch–Schönlein purpura** – This is more common in males aged 3–10 years – Usually, it occurs during the winter months – Often, it follows an upper-respiratory tract infection – Knee or ankle joint pain occurs in about 65% of patients – It is associated with a purpuric rash on the buttocks and thighs – Abdominal pain and hematuria occur in many children
A 5-year-old male child presents with a 1-day history of left-knee joint pain, associated with swelling and decreased range of movement, after a minor trauma. He had a history of excessive bleeding after circumcision	**Hemophilia** – In hemophilia, hemarthrosis may occur spontaneously or after a minor trauma – It usually starts in the ankle joint. The knees and elbows are also commonly affected in the older child and adolescent

(continued)

Table 2.10 (continued)

Short case scenarios	Diagnosis and special points in favor
A 10-year-old child presents with a 2-month history of migratory joint pain in combination with fever, weight loss, pallor, and petechiae	**Leukemia or lymphoma** – Arthralgia of leukemia or lymphoma is usually chronic and remitting – It is commonly associated with hepatomegaly or splenomegaly, petechiae, lymphadenopathy, pallor, and fever – The blood count may be normal at onset

History Station 2.31: Joint Pain

- **Identity:** Age, sex, ethnicity/race
- **Chief complaint:** Joint pain
- **History of present illness**
  1. Onset: Sudden or gradual
  2. Duration: Acute (e.g., trauma) or chronic (may suggest a serious underlying condition)
  3. Timing of the pain: Nighttime, daytime, or in the morning on arising
  4. Location and radiation of pain
  5. Number of joints involved
  6. Quality of pain
  7. Severity of pain: Does it interfere with normal activities?
  8. Progression over time: Static, increasing, or decreasing
  9. Intermittent or persistent, frequency of pain attacks, duration of each episode
  10. Associated symptoms: Warmth, redness, swelling, morning stiffness, decreased range of motion, limpness, refusal to walk, joint locking, joint giving way, fever, muscle weakness
  11. Aggravating and relieving factors: certain positions, activity (e.g., swimming), rest, heat, or medications
  12. Precipitating factors: A history of joint trauma, recent illnesses (e.g., gastroenteritis)
  13. Pre-existing joint disease
- **Past history**: History of trauma to the joint, prosthetic joint, previous arthritis, blood dyscrasias, psoriasis, sickle-cell anemia, diabetes, rickets, inflammatory bowel disease, celiac disease, chronic lung or cardiac disease with hypoxia, cystic fibrosis, uveitis, tuberculosis exposure, sexually transmitted disease exposure, surgery
- **Medication history:** Recent use of medications, corticosteroids, nonsteroidal anti-inflammatory drugs (NSAIDs), drug allergies
- **Immunization history:** Recent vaccination, such as *H. influenzae* immunization, MMR

Continued on the next page

- **Family history:** Family members with joint problems, sickle-cell anemia, hemophilia, psoriasis, inflammatory bowel disease, spondyloarthropathies, or uveitis
- **Social history:** Recent travel or tick bite, sanitation, overcrowded house, intravenous drug abuse, or child abuse
- **Review of systems:** Headache, fatigue, skin rash, chest pain, dyspnea, involuntary movements, dysuria, hematuria, bloody diarrhea, malaise, red eyes, or weight loss

Key Points 2.31

- Knowing the child's age is important (e.g., back pain in children younger than 5 years usually points to **a serious underlying pathology**, while in adolescents it is more likely to be due to **nonspecific musculoskeletal disorders**) [88].
- Fever, malaise, and weight loss may suggest **neoplasm** or **infection**.
- Pain that exacerbates at night is suggestive of **neoplasm** or **infection**.
- Migratory joint pain may be seen in a child with **acute rheumatic fever**, **post-streptococcal reactive arthritis**, **Henoch–Schönlein purpura**, or **childhood leukemia or lymphoma** [89].

References

1. Schwartz C. Dyspnea. In: Schwartz MW, Bell LM, Bingham PM, Chung EK, Friedman DF, Loomes KM, et al., editors. The 5-minute pediatric consult. 6th ed. Philadelphia: Lippincott Williams & Wilkins/Wolters Kluwer Business; 2012. p. 296–7.
2. Mayefsky JH. Dyspnea. In: Adam HM, Foy JM, editors. Signs and symptoms in pediatrics. Elk Grove Village, IL: The American Academy of Pediatrics; 2015. p. 235–45.
3. Stack AM. Etiology and evaluation of cyanosis in children. In: Teach SJ, Wiley JF, editors. UpToDate. 2017. http://www.uptodate.com/contents/etiology-and-evaluation-of-cyanosis-in-children. Accessed 12 Jan 2018.
4. Redjal N. Cough. In: Berkowitz CD, editor. Berkowitz's pediatrics: a primary care approach. 4th ed. Elk Grove Village, IL: The American Academy of Pediatrics; 2012. p. 503–8.
5. Boyer D, Zandieh S. Cough. In: Shah SS, Ludwig S, editors. Symptom-based diagnosis in pediatrics. 2nd ed. New York: McGraw-Hill; 2014. p. 89–116.
6. Ong T, Striegl A, Marshall SG. The respiratory system. In: Marcdante KJ, Kliegman RM, editors. Nelson essentials of pediatrics. 7th ed. Philadelphia: Elsevier Saunders; 2015. p. 455–80.
7. Goldfarb S, Brooks L. Wheezing. In: Schwartz MW, Bell LM, Bingham PM, Chung EK, Friedman DF, Loomes KM, et al., editors. The 5-minute pediatric consult. 6th ed. Philadelphia: Lippincott Williams & Wilkins/Wolters Kluwer Business; 2012. p. 948–9.
8. Vicencio AG, Needleman JP. Wheezing. In: Adam HM, Foy JM, editors. Signs and symptoms in pediatrics. Elk Grove Village, IL: The American Academy of Pediatrics; 2015. p. 987–96.

 9. Haferbacker DR. Wheezing. In: Shah SS, Ludwig S, editors. Symptom-based diagnosis in pediatrics. 2nd ed. New York: McGraw-Hill; 2014. p. 1–32.
10. Sidwell RU, Thomson MA. Easy pediatrics. Boca Raton, FL: CRC Press; 2011.
11. Miall L, Rudolf M, Smith D. Pediatrics at a glance. 3rd ed. Chichester: Wiley; 2012.
12. Chin-Sang S. Emergency management. In: Engorn B, Flerlage J, editors. The Harriet Lane handbook: a manual for pediatric house officers. 20th ed. Philadelphia: Elsevier Saunders; 2015. p. 3–18.
13. Stead LG, Stead SM, Kaufman MS. First aid for the pediatrics clerkship: a student to student guide. 2nd ed. Boston: McGraw-Hill; 2004.
14. Schneider DS. Chest pain. In: Marcdante KJ, Kliegman RM, editors. Nelson essentials of pediatrics. 7th ed. Philadelphia: Elsevier Saunders; 2015. p. 487–8.
15. Doroshow RW. Chest pain. In: Berkowitz CD, editor. Berkowitz's pediatrics a primary care approach. 4th ed. Elk Grove Village, IL: The American Academy of Pediatrics; 2012. p. 549–54.
16. Bernstein D. History and physical examination. In: Kleigman RM, Stanton BF, Schor NF, St Geme III JW, Behrman RE, editors. Nelson textbook of pediatrics. 20th ed. Philadelphia: Elsevier; 2016. p. 2163–70.
17. Drucker N. Syncope. In: Schwartz MW, Bell LM, Bingham PM, Chung EK, Friedman DF, Loomes KM, et al., editors. The 5-minute pediatric consult. 6th ed. Philadelphia: Lippincott Williams & Wilkins/Wolters Kluwer Business; 2012. p. 802–3.
18. Shah SS. Syncope. In: Shah SS, Ludwig S, editors. Symptom-based diagnosis in pediatrics. 2nd ed. New York: McGraw-Hill; 2014. p. 453–70.
19. Inkelis SH, Buitenhuys C. Sore throat. In: Berkowitz CD, editor. Berkowitz's pediatrics a primary care approach. 4th ed. Elk Grove Village, IL: The American Academy of Pediatrics; 2012. p. 445–52.
20. Carlo VS. Earache. In: Schwartz MW, Bell LM, Bingham PM, Chung EK, Friedman DF, Loomes KM, et al., editors. The 5-minute pediatric consult. 6th ed. Philadelphia: Lippincott Williams & Wilkins/Wolters Kluwer Business; 2012. p. 300–1.
21. Greenes D. Evaluation of earache in children. In: Fleisher GR, Wiley JF, editors. UpToDate. 2017. https://www.uptodate.com/contents/evaluation-of-earache-in-children. Accessed 12 Jan 2018.
22. Graessle WR. Otitis media. In: Schwartz MW, Bell LM, Bingham PM, Chung EK, Friedman DF, Loomes KM, et al., editors. The 5-minute pediatric consult. 6th ed. Philadelphia: Lippincott Williams & Wilkins/Wolters Kluwer Business; 2012. p. 612–3.
23. Gerber ME. Otitis media. In: Green TP, Franklin WH, Tanz R, editors. Pediatrics just the facts. New York: McGraw-Hill; 2005. p. 527–30.
24. Kabra SK. Upper respiratory tract infections. In: Parthasarathy A, Gupta P, Nair M, Menon P, Agarwal RK, Sukumaran T, editors. IAP textbook of pediatrics. 5th ed. New Delhi: Jaypee Brothers Medical Publishers; 2013. p. 484–6.
25. Cho CS. Ear, painful. In: Zorc JJ, Alpern ER, Brown LW, Loomes KM, Marino BS, Mollen CJ, et al., editors. Schwartz's clinical handbook of pediatrics. 5th ed. Philadelphia: Lippincott Williams & Wilkins Business; 2013. p. 317–25.
26. Brugha R, Marlais M, Abrahamson E. Pocket tour pediatrics clinical examination. London: JP Medical; 2013.
27. Gershma G. Abdominal pain. In: Berkowitz CD, editor. Berkowitz's pediatrics a primary care approach. 4th ed. Elk Grove Village, IL: The American Academy of Pediatrics; 2012. p. 713–8.
28. Gershma G. Vomiting. In: Berkowitz CD, editor. Berkowitz's pediatrics a primary care approach. 4th ed. Elk Grove Village, IL: The American Academy of Pediatrics; 2012. p. 679–83.
29. Aronson PL. Vomiting. In: Shah SS, Ludwig S, editors. Symptom-based diagnosis. New York: McGraw-Hill; 2014. p. 55–88.
30. Ulshen MH, McGreal N. Vomiting. In: Adam HM, Foy JM, editors. Signs and symptoms in pediatrics. Elk Grove Village, IL: The American Academy of Pediatrics; 2015. p. 971–7.

31. World Health Organization. IMCI handbook: integrated management of childhood illness. World Health Organization; 2005. http://www.who.int/maternal_child_adolescent/documents/9241546441/en/. Accessed 12 Dec 2017.
32. Gershman G. Diarrhea. In: Berkowitz CD, editor. Berkowitz's pediatrics a primary care approach. 4th ed. Elk Grove Village, IL: The American Academy of Pediatrics; 2012. p. 699–703.
33. Wiley CC. Diarrhea, acute. In: Zorc JJ, Alpern ER, Brown LW, Loomes KM, Marino BS, Mollen CJ, et al., editors. Schwartz's clinical handbook of pediatrics. 5th ed. Philadelphia: Lippincott Williams & Wilkins Business; 2013. p. 291–300.
34. Master CL. Diarrhea. In: Shah SS, Ludwig S, editors. Symptom-based diagnosis in pediatrics. 2nd ed. New York: McGraw-Hill; 2014. p. 429–52.
35. Grossman A. Diarrhea, chronic. In: Zorc JJ, Alpern ER, Brown LW, Loomes KM, Marino BS, Mollen CJ, et al., editors. Schwartz's clinical handbook of pediatrics. 5th ed. Philadelphia: Lippincott Williams & Wilkins Business; 2013. p. 301–10.
36. Rashid M. Evaluating gastrointestinal symptoms. In: Goldbloom RB, editor. Pediatric clinical skills. 4th ed. Philadelphia: Elsevier Saunders; 2011. p. 160–75.
37. Elizabeth K, Albright MD. Current clinical strategies pediatric history and physical examination. 4th ed. Laguna Hills, CA: Current Clinical Strategies Publishing; 2003.
38. Fiorino KN. Constipation. In: Zorc JJ, Alpern ER, Brown LW, Loomes KM, Marino BS, Mollen CJ, et al., editors. Schwartz's clinical handbook of pediatrics. 5th ed. Philadelphia: Lippincott Williams & Wilkins Business; 2013. p. 241–50.
39. Kahana DD, Gershman G. Constipation. In: Berkowitz CD, editor. Berkowitz's pediatrics a primary care approach. 4th ed. Elk Grove Village, IL: The American Academy of Pediatrics; 2012. p. 705–11.
40. Davey BT. Deja review pediatrics. New York: McGraw-Hill; 2008.
41. Belamarich PF. Constipation. In: Adam HM, Foy JM, editors. Signs and symptoms in pediatrics. Elk Grove Village, IL: The American Academy of Pediatrics; 2015. p. 119–33.
42. Avner JR. Gastrointestinal hemorrhage. In: Adam HM, Foy JM, editors. Signs and symptoms in pediatrics. Elk Grove Village, IL: The American Academy of Pediatrics; 2015. p. 395–407.
43. Gershman G. Gastrointestinal bleeding. In: Berkowitz CD, editor. Berkowitz's pediatrics a primary care approach. 4th ed. Elk Grove Village, IL: The American Academy of Pediatrics; 2012. p. 691–7.
44. Goel KM, Carachi R, Bhutta AZ. Gastroenterology and hepatology. In: Goel KM, Gupta DK, editors. Hutchison's pediatrics. 2nd ed. New Delhi: Jaypee Brothers Medical Publishers; 2012. p. 121–56.
45. Karjoo S, Liacouras CA. Gastrointestinal bleeding, lower. In: Zorc JJ, Alpern ER, Brown LW, Loomes KM, Marino BS, Mollen CJ, et al., editors. Schwartz's clinical handbook of pediatrics. 5th ed. Philadelphia: Lippincott Williams & Wilkins Business; 2013. p. 366–77.
46. Hsu EK. Jaundice. In: Zorc JJ, Alpern ER, Brown LW, Loomes KM, Marino BS, Mollen CJ, et al., editors. Schwartz's clinical handbook of pediatrics. 5th ed. Philadelphia: Lippincott Williams & Wilkins Business; 2013. p. 475–84.
47. Rose SR. Jaundice. In: Shah SS, Ludwig S, editors. Symptom-based diagnosis in pediatrics. 2nd ed. New York: McGraw-Hill; 2014. p. 375–402.
48. Pan DH, Rivas Y. Jaundice. In: Adam HM, Foy JM, editors. Signs and symptoms in pediatrics. Elk Grove Village, IL: The American Academy of Pediatrics; 2015. p. 581–95.
49. Ambalavanan N, Carlo WA. Jaundice and hyperbilirubinemia in the newborn. In: Kleigman RM, Stanton BF, Schor NF, St Geme III JW, Behrman RE, editors. Nelson textbook of pediatrics. 20th ed. Philadelphia: Elsevier Inc; 2016. p. 871–5.
50. Ruebner R, Pradhan M. Hematuria. In: Zorc JJ, Alpern ER, Brown LW, Loomes KM, Marino BS, Mollen CJ, et al., editors. Schwartz's clinical handbook of pediatrics. 5th ed. Philadelphia: Lippincott Williams & Wilkins Business; 2017. p. 414–23.
51. Reidy KJ, Rio MD. Hematuria. In: Adam HM, Foy JM, editors. Signs and symptoms in pediatrics. Elk Grove Village, IL: The American Academy of Pediatrics; 2015. p. 471–7.
52. Pan CG, Avner ED. Clinical evaluation of the child with hematuria. In: Kleigman RM, Stanton BF, Schor NF, St Geme III JW, Behrman RE, editors. Nelson textbook of pediatrics. 20th ed. Philadelphia: Elsevier Inc; 2016. p. 2494–6.

53. Valentini RP. Evaluation and management of edema in children. In: Mattoo TK, Kim MS, editors. UpToDate. 2017. http://www.uptodate.com/contents/evaluation-and-management-of-edema-in-children. Accessed 12 Jan 2018.

54. VanDeVoorde R. Edema. In: Zorc JJ, Alpern ER, Brown LW, Loomes KM, Marino BS, Mollen CJ, et al., editors. Schwartz's clinical handbook of pediatrics. 5th ed. Philadelphia: Lippincott Williams & Wilkins Business; 2013. p. 326–34.

55. Bichet DG. Diagnosis of polyuria and diabetes insipidus. In: Sterns RH, Emmett M, Forman JP, editors. UpToDate. 2017. http://www.uptodate.com/contents/diagnosis-of-polyuria-and-diabetes-insipidus. Accessed 12 Jan 2018.

56. Sampson M. Urinary frequency and polyuria. In: Zorc JJ, Alpern ER, Brown LW, Loomes KM, Marino BS, Mollen CJ, et al., editors. Schwartz's clinical handbook of pediatrics. 5th ed. Philadelphia: Lippincott Williams & Wilkins Business; 2013. p. 818–24.

57. Svoren BM, Jospe N. Type 1 diabetes mellitus (immune-mediated). In: Kleigman RM, Stanton BF, Schor NF, St Geme III JW, Behrman RE, editors. Nelson textbook of pediatrics. 20th ed. Philadelphia: Elsevier; 2016. p. 2763–90.

58. Haymond MW. Clinical features and diagnosis of diabetic ketoacidosis in children. In: Wolfsdorf JI, Hoppin AG, editors. UpToDate. 2017. http://www.uptodate.com/contents/clinical-features-and-diagnosis-of-diabetic-ketoacidosis-in-children. Accessed 12 Jan 2018.

59. Langdon DR. Diabetic ketoacedosis. In: Schwartz MW, Bell LM, Bingham PM, Chung EK, Friedman DF, Loomes KM, et al., editors. The 5-minute pediatric consult. 6th ed. Philadelphia: Lippincott Williams & Wilkins/Wolters Kluwer Business; 2012. p. 272–3.

60. Toy EC, Yetman RJ, Girardet RG, Hormann MD, Lahoti SL, McNeese MC, et al. Case files pediatrics. 3rd ed. New York: McGraw-Hill; 2009.

61. Ludwig S, Brandon CK. Poor weight gain. In: Shah SS, Ludwig S, editors. Symptom-based diagnosis in pediatrics. 2nd ed. New York: McGraw-Hill; 2014. p. 147–70.

62. Racine AD. Failure to thrive: pediatric undernutrition. In: Adam HM, Foy JM, editors. Signs and symptoms in pediatrics. Elk Grove Village, IL: The American Academy of Pediatrics; 2015. p. 301–15.

63. Huff KR. Headaches. In: Berkowitz CD, editor. Berkowitz's pediatrics a primary care approach. 4th ed. Elk Grove Village, IL: The American Academy of Pediatrics; 2012. p. 743–7.

64. Abend NS, Younkin D. Headache. In: Zorc JJ, Alpern ER, Brown LW, Loomes KM, Marino BS, Mollen CJ, et al., editors. Schwartz's clinical handbook of pediatrics. 5th ed. Philadelphia: Lippincott Williams & Wilkins Business; 2013. p. 404–13.

65. Wayman KA, Klein BC. Headache. In: Schwartz MW, Bell LM, Bingham PM, Chung EK, Friedman DF, Loomes KM, et al., editors. The 5-minute pediatric consult. 6th ed. Philadelphia: Lippincott Williams & Wilkins/Wolters Kluwer Business; 2012. p. 390–1.

66. Mikati MA, Hani AJ. Seizures in childhood. In: Kleigman RM, Stanton BF, Schor NF, St Geme III JW, Behrman RE, editors. Nelson textbook of pediatrics. 20th ed. Philadelphia: Elsevier; 2016. p. 2823–57.

67. Schiller JH, Shellhaas RA. Neurology. In: Marcdante KJ, Kliegman RM, editors. Nelson essentials of pediatrics. 7th ed. Philadelphia: Elsevier Saunders; 2015. p. 612–49.

68. Waldman AT. Seizures. In: Shah SS, Ludwig S, editors. Symptom-based diagnosis in pediatrics. 2nd ed. New York: McGraw-Hill; 2014. p. 471–97.

69. Migita R. Etiology and evaluation of the child with muscle weakness. In: Woodward GA, Wiley JF, editors. UpToDate. 2017. http://www.uptodate.com/contents/etiology-and-evaluation-of-the-child-with-muscle-weakness. Accessed 12 Jan 2018.

70. Brown LW. Paraplegia. In: Zorc JJ, Alpern ER, Brown LW, Loomes KM, Marino BS, Mollen CJ, et al., editors. Schwartz's clinical handbook of pediatrics. 5th ed. Philadelphia: Lippincott Williams & Wilkins Business; 2013. p. 614–23.

71. Abend NS. Coma. In: Zorc JJ, Alpern ER, Brown LW, Loomes KM, Marino BS, Mollen CJ, et al., editors. Schwartz's clinical handbook of pediatrics. 5th ed. Philadelphia: Lippincott Williams & Wilkins Business; 2013. p. 228–40.

72. Michelson D, Thompson L, Williams E. Evaluation of stupor and coma in children. In: Patterson MC, Wilterdink JL, Armspy C, editors. UpToDate. 2017. http://www.uptodate.com/contents/evaluation-of-stupor-and-coma-in-children. Accessed 12 Jan 2018.

73. Shah KN. Rash. In: Shah SS, Ludwig S, editors. Symptom-based diagnosis in pediatrics. 2nd ed. New York: McGraw-Hill; 2014. p. 223–56.

74. Krowchuk D. Rash. In: Adam HM, Foy JM, editors. Signs and symptoms in pediatrics. Elk Grove Village, IL: The American Academy of Pediatrics; 2015. p. 733–46.

75. Nield LS, Kamat D. Fever. In: Kleigman RM, Stanton BF, Schor NF, St Geme III JW, Behrman RE, editors. Nelson textbook of pediatrics. 20th ed. Philadelphia: Elsevier; 2016. p. 1277–9.

76. Balamuth F, Alpern ER. Fever. In: Zorc JJ, Alpern ER, Brown LW, Loomes KM, Marino BS, Mollen CJ, et al., editors. Schwartz's clinical handbook of pediatrics. 5th ed. Philadelphia: Lippincott Williams & Wilkins Business; 2013. p. 360–5.

77. Shah SS. Fever. In: Shah SS, Ludwig S, editors. Symptom-based diagnosis in pediatrics. 2nd ed. New York: McGraw-Hill; 2014. p. 279–304.

78. Baldwin KD, Wells W, Dormans JP. Clinical evaluation of the child. In: Kleigman RM, Stanton BF, Schor NF, St Geme III JW, Behrman RE, editors. Nelson textbook of pediatrics. 20th ed. Philadelphia: Elsevier; 2016. p. 3242–7.

79. Smith-Whitley K. Pallor. In: Zorc JJ, Alpern ER, Brown LW, Loomes KM, Marino BS, Mollen CJ, et al., editors. Schwartz's clinical handbook of pediatrics. 5th ed. Philadelphia: Lippincott Williams & Wilkins Business; 2013. p. 601–13.

80. Ludwig S, Brandon CK. Pallor. In: Shah SS, Ludwig S, editors. Symptom-based diagnosis in pediatrics. 2nd ed. New York: McGraw-Hill; 2014. p. 257–78.

81. McFarren AK, Levy AS. Anemia and pallor. In: Adam HM, Foy JM, editors. Signs and symptoms in pediatrics. Elk Grove Village, IL: The American Academy of Pediatrics; 2015. p. 47–62.

82. Mehta M. Malnutrition. In: Parthasarathy A, Gupta P, Nair M, Menon P, Agarwal RK, Sukumaran T, editors. IAP textbook of pediatrics. 5th ed. New Delhi: Jaypee Brothers Medical Publishers; 2013. p. 134–49.

83. Smith-Whitley K. Bleeding and purpura. In: Zorc JJ, Alpern ER, Brown LW, Loomes KM, Marino BS, Mollen CJ, et al., editors. Schwartz's clinical handbook of pediatrics. 5th ed. Philadelphia: Lippincott Williams & Wilkins Business; 2013. p. 193–208.

84. Tcheng WY. Bleeding disorders. In: Berkowitz CD, editor. Berkowitz's pediatrics a primary care approach. 4th ed. Elk Grove Village, IL: The American Academy of Pediatrics; 2012. p. 519–26.

85. Davidson J, Cleary AG, Bruce C. Disorders of bones, joints and connective tissues. In: Mcintosh N, Helms PJ, Smyth RL, Logan S, editors. Forfar and Arneil's textbook of pediatrics. 7th ed. Edinburgh: Elsevier Limited; 2008. p. 1385–446.

86. Armon K, Jackson L. Locomotion. In: Thalange N, Beach R, Booth D, Jackson L, editors. Pocket essentials of pediatrics. 2nd ed. Edinburgh: Elsevier Ltd; 2013. p. 41–57.

87. Seiden JA. Joint pain. In: Zorc JJ, Alpern ER, Brown LW, Loomes KM, Marino BS, Mollen CJ, et al., editors. Schwartz's clinical handbook of pediatrics. 5th ed. Philadelphia: Lippincott Williams & Wilkins Business; 2013. p. 504–16.

88. Aylor M. Back, joint and extremity pain. In: Shah SS, Ludwig S, editors. Symptom-based diagnosis in pediatrics. 2nd ed. New York: McGraw-Hill; 2014. p. 117–46.

89. Kimura Y, Southwood TR. Evaluation of the child with joint pain or swelling. In: Sundel R, TePas E, editors. UpToDate. 2017. http://www.uptodate.com/contents/evaluation-of-the-child-with-joint-pain-or-swelling. Accessed 12 Jan 2018.

90. Cvetnic WG, Pino E. USMLE step 2 CK pediatrics lecture notes. New York: Kaplan; 2013.

91. Boyer D, Kopel L. Chest pain. In: Shah SS, Ludwig S, editors. Symptom-based diagnosis in pediatrics. 2nd ed. New York: McGraw-Hill; 2014. p. 347–74.

92. Schroeder SA. Chest pain. In: Adam HM, Foy JM, editors. Signs and symptoms in pediatrics. Elk Grove Village, IL: The American Academy of Pediatrics; 2015. p. 111–8.

93. Wilkinson I, Subramanian GM. Headaches. In: South M, Isaacs D, editors. Practical pediatrics. 7th ed. Edinburgh: Elsevier; 2012. p. 625–35.

94. Hershey AD, Kabbouche MA, O'Brien HL. Headaches. In: Kleigman RM, Stanton BF, Schor NF, St Geme III JW, Behrman RE, editors. Nelson textbook of pediatrics. 20th ed. Philadelphia: Elsevier; 2016. p. 2863–74.

Part II

Examination of the Newborn and Older Child

Examination of the Newborn

3

There is nothing like a newborn baby to renew your spirit–
and to buttress your resolve to make the world a better place.

—*Virginia Clinton Kelley*

Contents

3.1   Introduction

- The neonatal period (the first 28 days after birth) is very important in human development. There is a high mortality rate during this period, especially within the first 24 h of life. Neonatal mortality rate (NMR), deaths during 28 days of life/1000 live births, is an important indicator of the health of a country. This rate constitutes up to 65% of the infant mortality rate (IMR). Therefore, more attention should be given to improving newborn care [1].

© Springer International Publishing AG, part of Springer Nature 2018
A. Qais Saadoon, *Essential Clinical Skills in Pediatrics*,
https://doi.org/10.1007/978-3-319-92426-7_3

- The performance of a comprehensive neonatal examination is extremely important and useful in identifying any congenital malformations or disorders and assessment of gestational age, vigor, and nutritional status. It can also prove reassuring to the baby's parents. Furthermore, it is considered a good opportunity for health promotion [2].
- Recording the information obtained from the neonatal examination is always important to establish a baseline upon which to build a picture of the child's development.
- Newborns should be examined comprehensively at least twice in the first few days of life [3, 4].
- A brief neonatal examination should be performed immediately after birth to assess the baby's general condition and to exclude any major congenital anomalies.
- A detailed routine physical examination should be performed for all newborns within the first 24 h of life and prior to discharge. This is an opportunity for early detection of any life-threatening disorders.
- In some countries, the recommendation is to perform the routine neonatal examination between 24 and 72 h of life to decrease the possibility of missing the diagnosis of some important conditions, such as congenital heart disease (CHD).
- Before the performance of the detailed routine neonatal physical examination, review relevant maternal history. Ask the mother about her health before and during the pregnancy, concentrating on medications she took during her pregnancy and illnesses from which she suffered, (e.g., gestational diabetes or hypertension). In addition to that, it is a good practice to talk with the mother about her labor and her feeling regarding the baby's wellness, concentrating on fetal health during the pregnancy and factors that may affect the current condition of the newborn. Important examples include breech presentation and threatened miscarriage [5].
- All maternal charts should be reviewed [6].
- While you are taking the birth history, observe the baby and surroundings for clues and important signs.
- Exclusive breastfeeding should be encouraged and discussed with parents before and during the antenatal period and soon after birth.
- The optimal time for an effective periodic examination of the newborn is a couple of hours after a feeding [3].
- As far as possible, carry out the examination in the presence of the parent(s). In fact, you should make a proactive effort to involve the baby's parents in his/her examination by encouraging them to undress their baby, hold him/her on their lap or the bed, and provide a stabilizing finger for him/her to grasp.
- If possible, while discarding the baby's diaper, make a note of whether the baby has had a bowel movement or passed urine.
- Wash your hands and dry them to avoid cold touch, and clean your stethoscope before the examination.

- Start the examination from head to toe in a well-lighted room.
- Keep the room temperature comfortably warm, with no running air conditioner or overhead fan that would cause a draft on the baby.
- Be flexible and patient during the examination, taking advantage of opportunities as they arise.
- Take the opportunity to auscultate the heart and the chest whenever the newborn is quiet.
- Avoid doing any potentially uncomfortable procedure, such as the hip examination, until the end of the examination. Such a procedure is likely to cause discomfort to the baby, making him/her cry and disrupt further examination.

3.2 Initial Brief Examination After Birth

- Newborns are usually stressed during parturition. Therefore, initial neonatal examination in the delivery room should be rapid and focus mainly on a careful inspection for major congenital anomalies, birth trauma, signs of depression or birth asphyxia, tone, activity, and level of consciousness.
- Note any pallor or cyanosis, as skin color is a good indicator for cardiac output.
- Monitor the temperature, auscultate the chest, and assess the heart rate and respiratory rate [7].
- Assess Apgar score and record it at 1 and 5 min (Table 3.1).
- Inspect the umbilical cord and determine the number of vessels. A normal umbilical cord should contain two arteries and one vein. The presence of only two vessels, one vein and one artery, may be associated with renal anomalies [8].
- Examine the placenta, as its size reflects intrauterine fetal growth. A small placenta is associated with a small newborn. Large edematous placentas are associated with the infant of a diabetic mother or erythroblastosis fetalis.
- Establish the baby's sex and exclude the presence of ambiguous genitalia.
- Establish anal patency and note the passage of urine and/or meconium.
- Dress the newborn and record all your findings.

Table 3.1 Apgar score [9, 10]

Element	Score		
	0 points	1 point	2 points
Appearance (color)	Blue, pale	Body pink, blue extremities	Pink all over
Pulse rate (heart rate)	Absent	<100 beats/min	>100 beats/min
Grimace (response to stimulation)	No response	Some movement	Cry, cough
Activity (muscle tone)	None, floppy	Some flexion	Active motion
Respiratory effort	Absent	Weak, irregular, gasps	Regular, strong cry

3.2.1 Apgar Score

- Apgar score refers to a rapid neonatal examination, which is carried out within the first few minutes of life to assess the newborn's progress or deterioration during the transition to extrauterine life [9].
- To assess the Apgar score, five parameters should be considered: the heart rate, breathing, muscle tone, color, and reflex irritability (response to the stimulation), each of these elements scoring 0–2 (see Table 3.1 and Box 3.1).
- Apgar score is usually assessed at 1 and 5 min after birth, but assessment of Apgar score at 10 min is sometimes needed (if the 5-minute Apgar score is below 7) [7].
- Healthy newborns commonly score 7 at 1 min, 8 at 5 min, and 10 at 10 min.
- If the Apgar score is less than 7, then the baby should be resuscitated, and the score should be calculated every 5 min until normal or for up to 20 min of life [10].

Box 3.1: Interpretation of 1-min Apgar Score [3, 10]

- From 0 to 3 indicates severe birth asphyxia; it requires immediate resuscitation and care in the NICU.
- From 4 to 6 indicates moderate birth asphyxia and requires close observation.
- From 8 to 10 indicates excellent condition (no birth asphyxia).

Notes 3.1

- In the first minute of life, if resuscitation is necessary (such as absence of a spontaneous cry or when the baby is cyanotic and floppy), resuscitation should be started immediately, regardless of the 1-minute Apgar score [3, 10].

3.3   Routine Examination of the Newborn Infant

Examination Station 3.1: Routine Examination of the Newborn Infant

At the start, consider all recommendations listed in the introduction of this chapter.

1. **General Observation and Assessment**
   - Appearance and general wellness
   - Level of alertness and activity
   - Dysmorphic features
   - Posture and movements

Continued on the next page

- Nutritional status assessment and anthropometric measurements
- Maturity and gestational age assessment
- Cry
- Vital signs

2. **Skin**
   - Inspection: Color, rash, or birthmarks
   - Palpation: Texture, turgor, and edema

3. **Head and Face**
   - Shape and size of the head, fontanels, and sutures
   - Facial dysmorphism, chin size
   - Eyes:
     - Size, position, symmetry, movement, red reflex, and discharge
   - Ears:
     - Size, position, and formation
   - Nose:
     - Patency, abnormalities (such as choanal atresia)
   - Mouth:
     - Size, other abnormalities (such as cleft lip/palate), and neonatal teeth

4. **Neck**
   - Swellings, edema, or webbing

5. **Arms and Hands**
   - Palsy, palmar creases, extra digit, and other abnormalities

6. **Chest**
   - Inspection, palpation, percussion, and auscultation

7. **Heart**
   - Inspection, palpation, and auscultation

8. **Abdomen**
   - Inspection, palpation, and auscultation

9. **Genitalia and Anus**
   - Inspection: malformations, ambiguous genitalia
   - Male newborn:
     - Penis, scrotum, testes (ensure both are fully descended)
   - Female newborn:
     - Labia minora and majora, vaginal and urethral opening, and hymen
   - Anus: Inspect its position and patency.

10. **Legs and Feet**
    - Inspection: Watch joint movements, deformities (such as clubfoot).
    - Count the toes, looking for any extra digit.
    - Elicit grasp reflex.

11. **Neurologic Examination**
    - Inspection: Movement and posture
    - Tone

Continued on the next page

- Reflexes:
  - Tendon reflexes, primitive reflexes
- Cranial nerve palsies
- Sensation: Observe reaction to touch, no pinprick used.
- Crude assessment of hearing and vision

12. **Spine and Sacrum**
  - Inspection: Any midline defect, tufts of hair, sinuses, or pits in the natal cleft may suggest spina bifida.
  - Palpation: Dimple or midline swelling

13. **Hips**
  - Inspection: Any asymmetrical skin creases or asymmetry of limb length
  - Examinations to detect developmental dysplasia of the hip (DDH)
    - Barlow test and Ortolani test

14. **Completing the Examination**
  - Take the temperature.
  - Measure the blood pressure.
  - Dress the baby and thank the parents.
  - Wash your hands.
  - Record your findings.

3.3.1 General Observation and Assessment

- Observe the general wellness of the newborn and note whether he/she looks well or ill.
- Assess his/her level of alertness and activity, as well as the general muscle tone.
- Note any dysmorphic features.
- Observe the baby's posture and movements.
  - Normally, the full-term newborn is in the fetal position, abducts and partially flexes his/her hips, flexes the knees, adducts his/her arms, and flexes them at the elbow.
  - A frog-like posture with very little spontaneous limb movement may suggest a hypotonia with lower motor neuron lesion in a term newborn. In a preterm newborn, a frog-like posture is normal [11].
- Nutritional status assessment and anthropometric measurements:
  - Note facial fullness, prominence of ribs with intercostal spaces, buttocks shape, as well as the skin and subcutaneous tissue over the thighs.
  - Weigh the baby, and measure his/her length as well as head circumference (i.e., occipitofrontal circumference, OFC), plotting these parameters on a standard growth chart appropriate to the baby's age and sex.

Notes 3.2

- All delivery rooms should have electronic weighing scales measuring to the nearest gram, and weight should be recorded in four digits (i.e., 3500 g not 3.5 kg).
- The birth weight of a normal newborn ranges between 2500 and 4500 g (median measurement is 3500 g) [5, 12].
- The normal head circumference of a term newborn should be between 33.5 and 37 cm (median measurement is 35 cm) [5, 12].
- The normal length of a full-term newborn is between 48 and 53.5 cm (median measurement is 50 cm) [5, 12].

Notes 3.3

- The first day of the last menstrual period and early antenatal ultrasound scans are useful for determination of the gestational age of a newborn. However, when these indicators are not available or there is doubt about the newborn's maturity, gestational age can be assessed in the first few days of life by the application of detailed systems designed for evaluating and scoring the gestational age of the newborn (e.g., the Dubowitz/Ballard Examination for Gestational Age). These systems depend on postnatal physical characteristics and neurologic development in the assessment of gestational age. It takes considerable experience and skill in practice to use them effectively and get accurate results [3, 4].

- Assess the newborn's maturity and gestational age using a Dubowitz/Ballard score.
- Newborns can be classified by gestational age or birth weight (see Table 3.2).
- There are many signs in the neonatal physical examination that help you to determine whether a newborn is full-term or preterm (see Table 3.3).

Table 3.2 Classification of newborns by gestational age or birth weight [6, 7]

Type	Gestational age	Type	Birth weight (g)
Term newborn	37–41 completed weeks of gestation	Normal birth weight	≥2500
Post-term, postmature newborn	≥42 completed weeks of gestation	Low birth weight (LBW)	<2500
Preterm newborn	<37 completed weeks of gestation	Very low birth weight (VLBW)	<1500
Extremely preterm	<28 completed weeks of gestation	Extremely low birth weight (ELBW)	<1000

Table 3.3 Some clinical differences between full-term and extremely preterm newborns [3, 22]

Element	Full-term newborn	Extremely preterm newborn
Posture	Flexed posture	Extended posture
Limb movements	Smooth	Jerky
Cry	Loud	Faint
Skin	Thick, pale-pink color	Very thin, gelatinous, dark-red color
Planter surface	Has deep creases crisscrossing the sole of the foot from the ball to the heel	The sole is smooth and deep creases are not present
Ears	Well-formed, pinna is firm, immediate recoil	Less well-formed, pinna is soft, no recoil
Genitalia, male	The scrotum has rugae, and the testes are entirely descended	The scrotum is smooth, and the testes are undescended
Genitalia, female	The labia majora entirely cover the clitoris and obscure the labia minora	The labia majora are widely seperated, the clitoris is prominent, and the labia minora are protruding
Breast	One or both nodules more than 1 cm	No breast tissue palpable

- Listen to the baby's cry, as it may provide a diagnostic clue (see Box 3.2).
  - Babies cry when they are hungry, uncomfortable, or disturbed.
  - The cry of a newborn is vigorous.

Box 3.2: The Baby's Cry [3, 13]

- A low-pitched and husky cry may suggest hypothyroidism.
- A high-pitched and shrill cry is suggestive of central nervous system abnormalities.
- A hoarse cry may point to vocal cord injury or congenital hypothyroidism.
- A weak cry may suggest sepsis or neuromuscular disease.
- A crowing cry suggests a laryngeal narrowing.

- **Vital Signs**
  - In a calm baby, assess the heart rate and check the respiratory rate by counting abdominal movements for 1 full minute.
  - Measurement of blood pressure and temperature may be uncomfortable for the baby. These should be left until last, if possible.
  - To know the normal ranges of the full-term newborn's vital signs, see Box 3.3.
  - Monitor oxygen saturation in all ill newborns (see Box 3.4).

Box 3.3: Normal Ranges of the Full-Term Newborn's Vital Signs [5, 6, 8, 12]

- Heart rate ranges between 100 and 160 beats per minute but may drop to 80 beats per minute during sleep.
- Respiratory rate ranges between 30 and 60 breaths per minute at rest.
- Systolic blood pressure on the first day of life ranges between 50 and 70 mmHg.
- Core temperature ranges from 36.7 °C to 37.3 °C. Temperature below 36.5 °C points to hypothermia, which should be a matter of concern.

Box 3.4: Pulse Oximetry [1]

- Pulse oximetry is a part of routine physical examination of the newborn to rule out critical congenital heart disease.
- In a normal term newborn, SpO_2 should be ≥95% after the first 24 h of life. This is 99% sensitive and specific in excluding critical congenital heart disease.
- By 24 h of life, all newborns with SpO_2 < 95% in the lower extremities should be evaluated carefully to rule out critical congenital heart disease.
- The difference of more than 10% of (SpO_2) between preductal (right upper extremity) and postductal (lower extremity) may suggest right-to-left shunt across the patent ductus arteriosus (PDA).
- During the first 10 min of life, preductal SpO_2 may fluctuate between 60 and 95%; this is considered normal.

3.3.2   Skin

- Inspection:
  - Observe for mild skin cracking and peeling in the post-term newborn and for relatively red skin and lanugo hair (fine hair) in the preterm newborn. Look for any bruising, petechia, or meconium staining.
  - Color:
    Observe the baby carefully, noting whether he/she is jaundiced; cyanotic (acrocyanosis, i.e., cyanosis of the hands and feet, is common on the first day of life, and it is of little significance in an otherwise normal newborn); pale; plethoric (as in small for gestational age or infant of a diabetic mother) [3].
  - Skin rash:
    Erythema toxicum neonatorum: Benign white, yellow pinpoint papules or vesicles at the center of red macules usually appear on the baby's trunk at 1–3 days of age and fade spontaneously within 1 week [4].

Milia: Small (1–2 mm) pearly white papules appear mainly on the face. They may present at birth and resolve spontaneously during the first 6 months of life.
- Birthmarks:
  Mongolian spots are gray-blue, macular, bruise-like birthmarks that may appear over the child's lower spine or buttocks and fade spontaneously, usually over the first year of life.
  Café au lait spots are light-brown macules that may occur in isolation or in association with a syndrome, especially when they are large and multiple (e.g., neurofibromatosis 1).
  Hemangiomas are common benign vascular tumors which may be superficial deep, or mixed.
  Port-wine stain (nevus flammeus) is a red/purple flat skin lesion that presents from birth and may thicken and become deeper in color with time. It may be associated with intracranial vascular malformation leading to Sturge-Weber syndrome [13].
  Nevus simplex (salmon patch) is a pale-pink macular birthmark that may present at birth on the baby's neck nape (known popularly as a stork bite), eyelids, or forehead. These birth marks usually resolve spontaneously over few months to years, except for those on the nape of neck, which tend to persist throughout life [4, 13].
- Palpation:
  - Palpate the skin texture and turgor.
  - Examine for edema:
    Generalized edema may suggest prematurity, congenital nephrosis, hypoproteinemia secondary to severe erythroblastosis fetalis, or nonimmune hydrops [1].
    Edema may cause absence of normal fine wrinkles usually found in the skin of a newborn's fingers or toes.

3.3.3 Head and Face

- Carefully inspect the baby's head, looking for:
  - The shape and size of the head.
  - Local trauma (e.g., minor scalp abrasions).
  - Cephalhematoma: A subperiosteal hemorrhage that does not extend across suture lines. It may take 3 weeks to 3 months to calcify and resolve, though it may lead to jaundice [5].
  - Caput succedaneum (molding): A soft, boggy swelling (scalp edema) that may extend across suture lines. It occurs secondary to pressure over the baby's skull during delivery. It is more common than cephalhematoma and usually disappears spontaneously within 1–4 days [4, 14].
  - Look at the baby's face, noting any:
    Swelling, forceps marks, or bruising (this may result from instrumental delivery).
    Dysmorphic features.

Facial asymmetry, which may suggest a transient facial nerve palsy.
– Note the chin size, excluding any abnormalities, e.g., micrognathia (underdeveloped jaw).
• Palpate the anterior and posterior fontanels, and assess their tension (the child should be examined in sitting position or being held upright) (see Box 3.5).
• Palpate the sutures, whether overlapping, prematurely fused (craniosynostosis), or widely separated, as in hydrocephalus [4, 15].
• Measure the head circumference of the newborn.

Box 3.5: The Fontanels

• The fontanels are membrane-covered openings in the baby's skull where the bones have not fused together yet.
• The anterior fontanel is large (varies greatly in size, measures 2–3 cm in diameter at birth) and closes between 9 and 18 months of age, while the posterior fontanel is small (<1 cm in diameter) and closes by 2 months of age (see Fig. 3.1) [15, 16].
• A depressed anterior fontanel is suggestive of dehydration, while a bulging fontanel is suggestive of increased intracranial pressure [15].

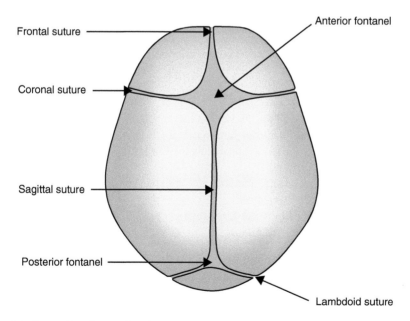

Fig. 3.1 Fontanels and suture lines in a newborn's skull

Eyes
- Inspect the newborn's eyes, observing the size, position, symmetry, and movements.
- Look at eyeballs, eyelids, eyelashes, and eyebrows, noting any abnormality, such as hypertelorism, subconjunctival hemorrhage, ptosis, or eyelid edema.
- Gently retract the lower eyelid and inspect the sclera for jaundice or any other abnormalities.
- Check for signs of infection, such as eye discharge.

Key Points 3.1

- Incomplete drainage of the lacrimal duct may lead to accumulation of lacrimal fluid—a common observation in newborns. It may be associated with secondary bacterial infection. However, the presence of a large amount of purulence should lead to consideration of a specific type of infection (e.g., gonococcal ophthalmia) [17].
- Squint is common in newborns, but only a few cases are paralytic and usually due to VI cranial nerve palsy [17].

- Look at the pupils, noting their size, shape, and color, and exclude the presence of cataracts.
- Elicit the red reflex, using an ophthalmoscope. An absent or partly obscured red reflex requires performance of the former fundoscopic examination at the end of the examination, as this may indicate a cataract or retinoblastoma.
- If possible, palpate the baby's eyeballs for eye pressure, comparing one to the other.

Ears

- Note the shape, size, and position of the ears, excluding any abnormalities (e.g., low-set ear; when an imaginary horizontal line is drawn from the outer canthus to the ear, the top of the pinna falls below the line). A low-set ear may be hereditary or a sign of a syndrome.
- Look for the ears' maturity, and note any bruising, preauricular tags, cysts, pits (small holes), fissures, or sinuses.
- Inspect the external auditory meatus for patency.

Nose
- Look at the nose for size, shape, and symmetry (asymmetry may indicate nasal fracture), and observe any nasal discharge, which may suggest early congenital syphilis [8].
- Babies are obligate nose breathers until 3 months of life. Hence, you must check carefully for patency of both nostrils by occluding airflow from one nostril and observing airflow from the other. Moreover, look for choanal atresia [19].

Mouth
- Inspect the mouth, looking for any asymmetry, micrognathia (small lower jaw), cleft lip, cleft palate, bifid uvula, oral thrush, Epstein pearls, natal teeth, etc.
- Examine the tongue, noting its size, shape, color, and abnormalities (e.g., short lingual frenulum, cyanosis, or macroglossia).
- Palpate inside the mouth along the hard palate, using your clean little finger, to exclude any abnormalities (e.g., submucosal clefts); at the same time, check the sucking reflex.

3.3.4   Neck

- Inspect the baby's neck, looking for midline masses, clefts, lateral neck masses, or sinuses.
- Look for neonatal torticollis (head tilt, caused by shortening of the sternocleido-mastoid muscle, commonly due to a fibrous tumor over the muscle, the so-called sternomastoid tumor).
- Neck edema, webbing or redundant neck skin with a low posterior hairline, may suggest Turner syndrome [8, 20].

3.3.5   Arms and Hands

- Observe the shape, length, symmetry, and movement of the arms for signs of Erb's palsy or Klumpke's palsy.
- Inspect the newborn's hands, noting the number of palmar creases. Although it is found in 1–2% of the general population, a single palmar crease on both palms is often a feature of Down syndrome [11].
- Observe the fingers, checking their number, noting any abnormalities, such as short incurved fingers (clinodactyly, generally the fifth finger as in Down syndrome), increase in a number of fingers (polydactyly), or fused fingers (syndactyly).
- Elicit the grasp reflex.

3.3.6   Chest

Inspection
- Observe the color of the newborn's lips, mucous membranes, and skin, excluding any cyanosis. (Acrocyanosis is normal, while central cyanosis is pathologic.)
- Listen for any abnormal sounds; these may include grunting, stridor, or wheeze.
- Inspect the shape of the chest for any deformity, and notice any use of accessory muscles for respiration.
- Observe the pattern of the newborn's respiration; it is usually irregular, with relative tachypnea and alternating short pauses (periodic breathing). The breathing of a normal newborn is effortless and predominately diaphragmatic.

- Note any signs of respiratory distress, such as flaring of the alae nasi, or subcostal, intercostal, and sternal retractions.
- Count the respiratory rate in 1 full minute.
- Observe the breast tissue and nipple development, noting any extra nipple.

Palpation and Percussion
- Localize the apex beat; it may be shifted toward the collapsed lung and away from tension pneumothorax and diaphragmatic hernia.
- Palpate along the clavicles to exclude fractures, which may occur during delivery; also feel for any crepitus or swelling.
- Palpate the neck and chest for subcutaneous emphysema, which may suggest a pneumothorax or pneumomediastinum [20].
- Palpate the breast for any tenderness, which may suggest mastitis or breast abscess, especially if it is associated with asymmetry, induration, and erythema [1].
- Percussion has a little value in the respiratory examination of the newborn.

Auscultation
- Auscultate the chest anteriorly, laterally, and posteriorly, listening for air entry, the symmetry of breath sounds, and any additional sounds.

Key Points 3.2

- Hearing of bowel sounds in the chest may suggest a diaphragmatic hernia, especially if it is associated with a scaphoid (boat-shaped) abdomen [10].

3.3.7 Heart

Inspection
- Observe the color of the newborn, looking for any cyanosis.
- Note chest shape and any precordial bulge, and observe respiratory efforts.

Palpation
- Palpate the precordium for the apex beat (normally present at the fourth intercostal space in the left mid-clavicular line) [13].
- Feel for the thrill and left parasternal heave with the palm of your hand.
- Palpate for brachial, radial, and femoral pulses on both sides, as absence of the femoral pulse on either side is suggestive of coarctation of the aorta.

Auscultation
- Use both the bell and the diaphragm of your stethoscope to auscultate the newborn's heart at both the apex and the base.
- Measure the heart rate, and listen for the first heart sound at the apex and the second heart sounds at the base.
- Describe any pathological murmurs or additional sounds.

Clinical Tips 3.1

- In the sleeping baby, listen to the heart sounds before undressing. This will prevent his/her crying during your auscultation [11].
- The presence of a murmur in the first 24 h of life may be normal; it may reflect a closing ductus, or it may be functional, so it does not always indicate congenital heart disease. However, hearing a loud, coarse systolic murmur in the first 72 h of life may indicate obstruction [19].
- Obtaining the oxygen saturation in the lower extremities of a newborn with a cardiac murmur is a good practice. A saturation of more than 96% may exclude serious congenital heart disease. However, this is not a substitute for examination by a more senior pediatrician [15].

3.3.8   Abdomen

Inspection
- Observe the abdomen for distention. In general, a newborn's abdomen is often somewhat protuberant (particularly after a feeding).
- A scaphoid abdomen suggests congenital diaphragmatic hernia.
- Look for any visible bowel loops or rectus sheath diastasis.
- Inspect the umbilical stump (if present), looking for:
    - Any signs of infection (redness, abnormal odor, and discharge)
    - The three umbilical vessels (two arteries and one vein)
    - Umbilical granuloma
    - Umbilical hernia, gastroschisis, or omphalocele

Notes 3.4

- The umbilical cord is usually desiccated and separated spontaneously from the abdomen at the fourth or fifth day of life [17].

- Note any diaper dermatitis.
- Inspect the newborn's stool (if available).
- Carefully inspect the groin, looking for any inguinal hernia.
- A rectal examination is not routinely performed unless indicated [4].

Palpation
- With a warm right hand, perform both superficial and deep palpations of the newborn's abdomen.
- The tip of the spleen, the soft liver edge 1–2 cm below the right costal margin, and the lower poles of both kidneys can normally be palpated in a newborn [10].
- Palpation of the newborn's kidneys requires considerable practice. They can be examined by placing one of your hands under the upper lumbar region and pressing gently upward while palpating the kidney with the other hand. They can also be palpated by using the thumb and index finger, encircling the flank.
- Palpate for the bladder using your thumb, index, and second fingers. Start the palpation just below the umbilicus and move downward until you feel the bladder. The optimal time for bladder palpation is 15 min after feeding. A palpable bladder to the umbilicus may suggest a severe neural tube defect (NTD) or central nervous system (CNS) damage [13].

Auscultation
- Auscultation of the abdomen for bowel sounds is not a part of routine abdominal examination unless indicated [14].

3.3.9   Genitalia and Anus

- Carefully examine the genitalia of a male or female newborn, excluding any abnormalities (e.g., ambiguous genitalia).
- For a male newborn:
  - Inspect the penis, noting its size and shape, and excluding any hypospadias or other abnormalities.
  - Inspect the scrotum. You should see deep rugae.
  - Palpate the testes on both sides of the scrotal sac, ensuring their presence and confirming that their size is normal. If they are not present in the scrotal sac, palpate the inguinal area. Hydrocele or hernia should be noted.

Notes 3.5

- The penis is covered completely by foreskin, which cannot and should not be entirely retracted during penile examination [3].
- The urethral meatus is normally located at the tip of the glans; it may or may not be possible to see [3].
- The mean stretched length of a term newborn's penis is about 3.5 cm ± 0.7 [21].
- A unilateral undescended testis normally descends by 6 months of age. Hence, this does not require intervention before that time [15].
- A baby with bilateral undescended testes should be reviewed by a more senior pediatrician to confirm the diagnoses and conduct further investigations [15].
- The scrotum of a baby with undescended testes is usually underdeveloped.
- In a preterm baby, testes may be felt at a higher level in the inguinal canal.

- For a female newborn, inspect the external genitalia. In a normal full-term newborn, the labia majora are swollen and cover the labia minora and clitoris. Put your thumbs on the labia majora and push laterally, ensuring the patency of the urethral and vaginal opening and noting the size and color of the clitoris. Inspect the hymen, which may appear thick and may have a hymenal tag. A hymenal tag or vaginal skin tag may be normal, requiring no treatment.
- Observe the newborn's anus. It should be patent and in its normal location.

3.3.10 Legs and Feet

- Inspect the newborn's legs and feet, observing the movement of each joint and looking for symmetry, abnormalities, and deformities, such as talipes (clubfoot), or puffiness of the feet (as seen in Turner syndrome) [4].
- A mild or moderate bowing of the lower leg of a newborn is a minor variant.
- If you notice clubfoot, try to ascertain its type. The foot can be straightened in the case of postural type, while in the case of the fixed clubfoot, the curved shape of the foot cannot be straightened.
- Count the number of toes, noting any extra digits. A mild syndactyly of the second and third toes is a minor variant, not a minor anomaly [1].
- Ensure the presence of the toenails. Toenails often look ingrown in newborns. This is a normal finding and does not require any intervention [1, 17].
- Elicit the grasp reflex.

3.3.11 Neurologic Examination

- Start with inspection, observing **the posture** of the newborn. Normally, all extremities are flexed [20].
- Look for spontaneous **movements** of the baby. Make a note of the symmetry of his/her movements.
- Listen to the baby's cry and assess its quality.
- Assess **the tone** by observing the baby's resting posture and then performing the following tests:
  - *Scarf sign*
    To assess the upper extremity tone, pull the newborn's arm across his/her chest toward the opposite shoulder. Normally, the elbow should not reach the midline; in the case of hypotonia, the elbow will cross the midline.
  - *Pull to sit*
    Grasp the newborn's hands, and slowly pull him/her from the supine to the sitting position while you are observing his/her head. In the case of hypotonia, the head lags backward, and when an erect position is assumed, it drops forward, while in hypertonia, the baby's head is kept backward (see Fig. 3.2b) [11].
  - *Axillary (vertical) suspension*
    Hold the newborn's chest with your hands, and suspend the baby, lifting him/her in an upright position, while you are watching the legs.

A hypotonic baby tends to slip through your hands.

In the case of cerebral palsy or other causes of spasticity, you may see scissoring or hyperextension of the legs [13].

- *Ventral (horizontal) suspension*

   While the infant is prone, put your hand under his/her trunk, and gently lift the infant upward. Normally, the newborn extends the back and flexes the arms and knees, while lifting and rotating the head. A hypotonic infant will droop over your hands like a rag doll (see Fig. 3.2a) [13, 17].

   Look for the position of the baby's neck. An extended neck may indicate "cerebral irritation" or severe meningism.

- Palmar grasp and Moro reflexes are helpful in the assessment of proximal and distal muscle power.
- Tendon reflexes are not routinely elicited unless the newborn has neurological or muscular abnormalities.
- Elicit the primitive reflexes (see Table 3.4).
- The sensation can be assessed by applying gentle (not painful) stimuli and noting whether the baby withdraws from it or not. It is not part of a routine examination.
- Look for any signs of cranial nerve palsies, such as facial asymmetry (especially when crying), failure of eye closure, and feeding difficulty. These signs may suggest facial (CN VII) nerve palsy.

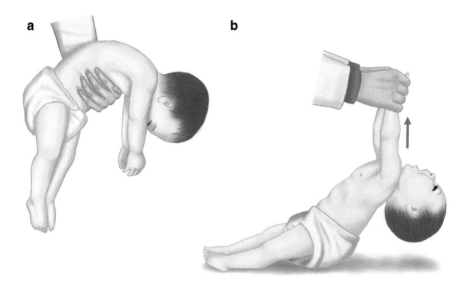

Fig. 3.2 Assessment of the baby's tone. (**a**) A "rag doll" flexion in ventral (horizontal) suspension (floppy infant). (**b**) Pulling the floppy infant from supine to a sitting position (the head lag continues even when the siting position is reached). ©Anwar Qais Saadoon

- Examine eyesight by observing the alert baby in both dark and bright areas. In a dark area, he/she may open eyes wide, while he/she closes them tightly in a bright area.
- Hearing can be tested crudely by observing the startle response to a sound. Universal newborn hearing screening by elicitation of brainstem auditory-evoked responses (BEAR) is routine in many countries [4, 7].

Table 3.4 The primitive reflexes [4, 10, 13, 20]

Reflex	Description	Age at appearance	Age at disappearance
Stepping	The infant steps up if he/she is held upright with the dorsum of the feet touching a flat surface	Birth	5 weeks–4 months
Galant	In ventral suspension, stroking the paravertebral region of the back will cause movement of the pelvis toward the stimulated side	Birth	2–6 months
Asymmetrical tonic neck response	Turning of the baby's head to the side while he/she is supine will cause extension of the arm and leg on the side toward which the head is turned and flexion of the arm and leg on the contralateral side (see Fig. 3.3a)	Birth, but fully developed by 1 month	3–6 months
Moro	Abduction and extension, followed by adduction and flexion, of the baby's arms symmetrically, when his/her head is dropped back suddenly from a semi-erect position onto the examiner's hand (see Fig. 3.3b)	Birth	3–6 months
Rooting	If you stroke the baby's cheek, he/she will open his/her mouth and turn toward the stimulus	Birth	4–6 months
Sucking	Gentle pressure on the hard palate produces a reflexive sucking	Birth	Becomes voluntary at 3–6 months
Palmar grasp	The baby's hand closes when the palm is stroked	Birth	4–6 months
Plantar (Babinski)	Stroking the lateral aspect of the sole of the foot with a firm object (beginning at the heal and extending to the base of the toes) produces dorsal flexion of the big toe and fanning of the other toes	Birth	12–18 months
Glabellar tap	A sharp tap on the glabella causes momentary closure of the eyes or blinking	Birth	Variable
Parachute	The baby's arms extend and his/her hands open up when he/she is brought rapidly down toward the floor while ventrally suspended	8–10 months	Never

Note: In certain neurological diseases, such as cerebral palsy, primitive reflexes persist beyond these age limits [13]

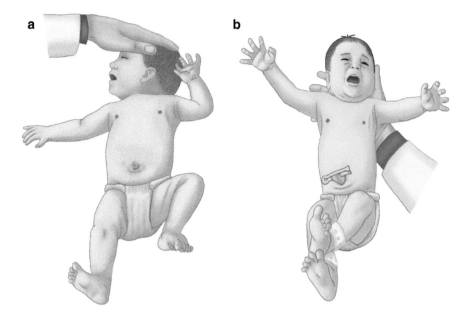

Fig. 3.3 The primitive reflexes. (**a**) Asymmetrical tonic neck response. (**b**) Moro (startle) reflex.
©Anwar Qais Saadoon

3.3.12 Spine and Sacrum

- With the baby prone, inspect the skin over the spine, looking for any skin changes or abnormalities (e.g., hyperpigmentation).
- Note any tufts of hair, sinuses, or deep sacral pits in the natal cleft. These signs may suggest a spina bifida [19].
- Note any deformities (e.g., kyphosis or scoliosis) [13].
- Run your finger along the newborn's spine to the occiput, palpating each spinal process and looking for any midline swelling or dimple. If present, a postanal dimple is of no significance. You should reassure the parents.

3.3.13 Hips

- Examination of the hips may upset the newborn. With this in mind, it is best left until last [18].
- The baby's diaper must be removed.
- Start with inspection of the thighs, looking for clinical signs that may suggest hip dislocation. Look for asymmetrical skin creases and asymmetry of limb length.
- Gently abduct the newborn's hips. The ability to perform a full abduction on both sides rules out hip dislocation [15].

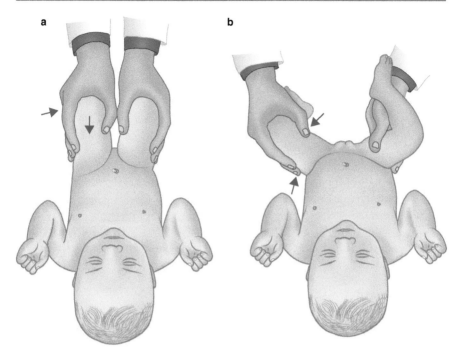

Fig. 3.4 Examination of the hip in newborns. (**a**) *Barlow test*. Check whether the hip can be dislocated posteriorly out of acetabulum by applying longitudinal pressure along the femoral shaft. (**b**) *Ortolani test*. Check whether the dislocated hip can be relocated back into acetabulum by lifting the head of the femur forward with your middle finger while you are abducting the thigh with your thumb

- Perform the Barlow and the Ortolani tests to rule out the presence of developmental dysplasia of the hip (DDH) (see Fig. 3.4a, b), which is more common in female newborns.
  - ***Barlow test***
    Here the femoral head is in place, but the hip is dislocatable posteriorly.
    Remove the baby's diaper, and put him/her in the supine position on a firm, flat surface.
    The newborn should be relaxed, if possible.
    Flex his/her knees at 90°, and adduct the hips until the knees touch each other in the midline.
    Place the tip of your middle finger over the greater trochanter of the femur, with your thumb on the internal side of the thigh over the medial condyle.
    Try to dislocate the hip posteriorly by applying longitudinal pressure along the femoral shaft (see Fig. 3.3a).
    A palpable "clunk" indicates the head of the femur has been dislocated, meaning a **positive Barlow test.**

- *Ortolani test*
  The aim of the Ortolani test is to relocate a hip that is already dislocated.
  Remove the baby's diaper and place him/her in the supine position on a firm surface.
  Begin with the baby's knees together and flex both knees and hips at 90°.
  Place the tip of your middle finger over the greater trochanter of the femur, with your thumb on the internal side of the thigh over the medial condyle.
  Attempt to lift the head of the femur forward with your middle finger while you are abducting the thigh with the thumb (see Fig. 3.4b).
  A palpable clunk (or an audible click) indicates **a positive Ortolani sign.** (The posteriorly dislocated femoral head is returning to the acetabulum.)
  Repeat the same maneuver on the other hip.
- Barlow and Ortolani tests are not reliable after the age of 6 weeks in discovering the developmental dysplasia of the hip due to increased muscle tone. After that time, a limited hip abduction is the only reliable clinical test to discover hip dislocation [13].

3.3.14   Completing the Examination

- Measure the baby's temperature in the axilla. If it is abnormal, measure the rectal temperature for confirmation.
- Check the blood pressure in all ill newborns and in those with heart murmur or heart failure [1, 16].
- Offer to dress the newborn, and address any questions the parents may have.
- Thank the parents and explain the next steps.
- Wash your hands.
- Record your findings.

References

1. Carlo WA. The newborn infant. In: Kleigman RM, Stanton BF, Schor NF, St Geme III JW, Behrman RE, editors. Nelson textbook of pediatrics. 20th ed. Philadelphia: Elsevier; 2016. p. 794–8.
2. Lissauer T, Sharkey D. Perinatal medicine. In: Lissauer T, Carroll W, editors. Illustrated textbook of pediatrics. 5th ed. Edinburgh: Elsevier; 2018. p. 142–65.
3. Howlett AA, Jangaard K. Evaluating the newborn: diagnostic approach. In: Goldbloom RB, editor. Pediatric clinical skills. 4th ed. Philadelphia: Elsevier Saunders; 2011. p. 38–55.
4. Becher JC, Lasing I. History, examination, basic investigations and procedures. In: Mcintosh N, Helms PJ, Smyth RL, Logan S, editors. Forfar and Arneil's textbook of pediatrics. 7th ed. Edinburgh: Elsevier; 2008. p. 115–58.
5. Sinha S, Miall L, Jardine L. Essential neonatal medicine. 5th ed. Chichester: Wiley; 2012.
6. Lissauer T, Fanaroff A. Neonatology at glance. 2nd ed. Chichester: Blackwell Publishing; 2011.

7. Stenson B, Turner S. Examination in specific situation: babies and children. In: Douglas G, Nicol F, Robertson C, editors. Macleod's clinical examination. 13th ed. Edinburgh: Elsevier; 2013. p. 355–78.

8. Rosenberg AA, Grover T. The newborn infant. In: Hay WW, Levin MJ, Abzug MJ, Deterding RR, editors. Current diagnosis and treatment pediatrics. 22th ed. New York: McGraw-Hill; 2014. p. 78–198.

9. Apgar V. A proposal for a new method of evaluation of the newborn infant. Curr Res Anesth Analg. 1953;32:260–7.

10. Sidwell RU, Thomson MA. Easy pediatrics. Boca Raton: CRC Press; 2011.

11. Brugha R, Marlais M, Abrahamson E. Pocket tour pediatrics clinical examination. London: JP Medical Ltd; 2013.

12. Vishnu Bhat B, Vani S, Chatterjee R, Gupte S. Neonatology. In: Gupte S, editor. The short textbook of pediatrics. 12th ed. New Delhi: Jaypee Brothers Medical Publishers; 2016. p. 267–330.

13. Stephenson T, Wallace H, Thomson A. Clinical pediatrics for postgraduate examination. 3rd ed. Elsevier Science: Edinburgh; 2002.

14. Narang M. Approach to practical pediatrics. 2nd ed. New Delhi: Jaypee Brothers Medical Publishers; 2011.

15. Goel KM, Carachi R. Pediatric history and examination. In: Goel KM, Gupta DK, editors. Hutchison's pediatrics. 2nd ed. New Delhi: Jaypee Brothers Medical Publishers; 2012. p. 1–17.

16. Szilagyi PG. Assessing children: infancy through adolescence. In: Bickley LS, Szilagyi PG, editors. Bates' guide to physical examination and history-taking. 11th ed. Philadelphia: Wolters Kluwer Health/Lippincott Williams & Wilkins; 2013. p. 765–891.

17. Gill D, O'Brien N. Pediatric clinical examination made easy. 6th ed. Edinburgh: Elsevier; 2017.

18. Newell SJ, Darling JC. Pediatrics lecture notes. 9th ed. Wiley: Chichester; 2014.

19. Noble JE. Neonatal examination and nursery visit. In: Berkowitz CD, editor. Berkowitz's pediatrics a primary care approach. 4th ed. Elk Grove Village, IL: American Academy of Pediatrics; 2012. p. 99–104.

20. Gowen CW. Fetal and neonatal medicine. In: Marcdante KJ, Kliegman RM, editors. Nelson essentials of pediatrics. 7th ed. Philadelphia: Elsevier; 2015. p. 186–233.

21. Elder JS. Anomalies of the penis and urethra. In: Kleigman RM, Stanton BF, Schor NF, St Geme III JW, Behrman RE, editors. Nelson textbook of pediatrics. 20th ed. Philadelphia: Elsevier; 2016. p. 2586–92.

22. Lissauer T, Sharkey D. Neonatal medicine. In: Lissauer T, Carroll W, editors. Illustrated textbook of pediatrics. 5th ed. Edinburgh: Elsevier; 2018. p. 166–93.

Examination of the Older Child

> *Accuracy of observation is the equivalent of accuracy of thinking.*
>
> *—Wallace Stevens*

Contents

© Springer International Publishing AG, part of Springer Nature 2018
A. Qais Saadoon, *Essential Clinical Skills in Pediatrics*,
https://doi.org/10.1007/978-3-319-92426-7_4

4.1   Introduction

- The examination of a pediatric patient is a challenge as its specifics vary with the child's age. In addition, children often do not like to be examined and, therefore, may often get upset. Understandably, in order to adequately examine a child and make an accurate diagnosis, you must develop your own technique and style for the examination. It should always be adapted to the situation and the child's age.
- The physical examination usually starts with the initial observation of the child at the moment of his/her entry into the consulting room. This initial observation, along with the taking of a thorough history, should guide you in performing an appropriate physical examination of the corresponding organ system. An aimless physical examination is unhelpful; it will only consume time and upset the child and his/her parents.
- The examination room should be clean, warm, and child-friendly, with good light (preferably natural light).
- Try to make the child cooperate with you through the following:
  - Greet him/her and the parents in a friendly way.
  - Explain gently to the child and the parents what you are going to do.
  - Always be relaxed and maintain a respectful manner and pleasant expression.
  - As far as possible, try to be confident but gentle while examining the child, and avoid any irritation or anything that may cause crying.

> *If a child cries when you examine it, then it's probably your fault.*
> *—John Apley*

- Start speaking with the parents first, with a calm and quiet voice and a friendly tone. This will give the child a chance to study you. In addition, try to make your movements gentle and unhurried, and avoid sudden movements.
- Examine the child with empathy, patience, and flexibility.
- Begin the examination at a non-threatening part of the body, such as the hands. In a younger child, try to examine the most critical areas (such as the heart and lungs) first, before he/she cries.
- Have toys, games, and books available in the consulting room, suitable for all ages.
- Play with the children. This may be helpful in getting their cooperation [1].

> *You can do anything with children if you only play with them.*
>
> —*Otto von Bismarck*

- Adapt your examination according to the child's age:
  - Examine infants in the first few months of life on the examination table, with a parent next to them.
  - Examine children from 3 months to 3 years of age on their mother's lap or over her shoulder.
  - Observe preschool children while they are playing, and examine them on the examination table or while standing.
  - School-age children and adolescents are often concerned about privacy. They may comply with a full adult style of physical examination on the examination table.
  - A teenage female should not be examined unless her mother or a female chaperone is present.
- Equipment, such as a stethoscope, otoscope, penlight, and tongue depressor should be at hand.
- Before starting the examination, follow the steps in Clinical Tips 4.1.

Clinical Tips 4.1

- Before starting the physical examination, take the following steps (mnemonic **WIPE**):
  - **W**ash your hands, then dry and warm them.
  - **I**ntroduce yourself to the child and parents after greeting them, then confirm the child's name and age, and explain what you are going to do.
  - Ask for **p**ermission to examine the child and place him/her in a suitable **p**osition, according to his/her age and the part of the body that you want to examine.
  - **E**xpose the area as needed for the examination (better to be performed by the child or by his/her parents), and **e**xamine from the right side of the patient.
- At the end of the examination, thank the child and parents, and wash your hands.

- Invasive and potentially discomforting procedures, as well as examination of threatening areas (e.g., the oral cavity and ears), should be left until later, at the end of the examination, as they may disturb further examination by making the child cry.
- For the purpose of this chapter, a detailed physical examination of each system will be described here separately. Nonetheless, in practice, your own examination should be guided by the patient's history and your initial observations.

4.2   General Inspection

- **Initial impression**
  - Is the child well or ill, smiling or miserable, playful or apathetic, comfortable or uncomfortable?
  - Note whether the child is lethargic, unconscious, irritable, apprehensive, hyperactive, etc.
  - Note any unusual behavior or parent–child interaction, and observe the reaction of the child to someone new entering the room (this may provide clues to the possibility of child abuse).

Clinical Tips 4.2

- Differentiate the tired child from one who is lethargic; the latter is difficult to arouse.
- Distinguish the truly irritable child from one who is cranky; the latter can easily be comforted [2].

- **Posture, gait, and movements**
  - Note any abnormal or unusual postures, such as scissoring of the legs or a windswept posture. Observe the child for abnormal gaits, such as a waddling gait (as in developmental dysplasia of the hip or Duchenne muscular dystrophy). Also note any involuntary movements, such as chorea or tics.
- **Body shape and dysmorphic features**
  - Inspect for any abnormal body shape and note the general body proportions.
  - Note any dysmorphic features which may suggest a genetic or teratogenic disorder, such as cleft lip or palate, epicanthal folds, low-set ears, etc.
- **Color and odor**
  - Note the skin color, whether it is yellow (jaundice, as in hepatitis or hemolytic anemia), blue (cyanosis, as in a patient with cyanotic congenital heart disease), or pale (pallor, as in an anemic child).
  - Smell for any abnormal odor, such as an **acetone smell**, as in a patient with diabetic ketoacidosis (DKA) or starvation, and **halitosis** (bad breath), as in gingivitis, stomatitis, or atrophic rhinitis.
- **Dress and hygiene:** These may give an idea about the social circumstances and the care that the child receives from the family, and they also may point to the state of mind in older children and adolescents [3].

- **Cry**
  - Listen to the cry of the child, whether it is normal, low, or high-pitched. A low-pitched cry may result from grave illness, generalized weakness, or respiratory muscle weakness, while a high-pitched cry may point to a serious condition, such as meningitis [4].

4.3   Assessment of Hydration Status

- Infants are at greater risk of dehydration than adults, for a variety of reasons. For example, they have high fluid intake needs in comparison to adults, and they have little or no control over fluid intake [1].
- Generally, hydration status can be assessed using the following parameters: General condition and level of consciousness, eyes, skin turgor, skin warmness and color, fontanels, tears, the degree of mouth and tongue dryness, breathing, capillary refill time, pulse rate and quality, urine output, and systolic blood pressure measurement.
- According to the clinical assessment, dehydrated children can be classified into those with **mild**, **moderate**, or **severe dehydration** [5, 6] (see Table 4.1).
- The World Health Organization (WHO) defines dehydration in children with diarrhea according to four parameters that classify children as having **no dehydration**, **some dehydration**, or **severe dehydration** (see Table 4.2). These classifications are very important in the treatment of children with diarrhea. There are specific diarrhea treatment plans (A, B, and C) adopted by the WHO; you should choose the most appropriate plan for each classification [10].

Table 4.1 Clinical assessment of hydration status in children [5–8]

Parameters	Mild dehydration	Moderate dehydration	Severe dehydration
General condition and level of consciousness	Well, alert	Unwell, restless, irritable, or deteriorating[a]	Unwell, apathetic, lethargic, or unconscious
Eyes	Normal	Slightly sunken[a]	Very sunken
Skin turgor	Normal (instant recoil)	Reduced[a]	Tenting
Skin	Warm	Cool and pale	Cold, mottled, cyanotic
Fontanel (infants)	Flat	Slightly sunken	Very sunken
Tears	Normal	Normal to decreased	Absent
Mucous membranes	Moist or slightly dry	Dry	Parched/cracked
Breathing	Normal	Deep, rate may be fast[a]	Deep, fast, or absent
Capillary refill	<2 s	Prolonged (2–3 s)	Very delayed (>3 s)

(continued)

Table 4.1 (continued)

Parameters	Mild dehydration	Moderate dehydration	Severe dehydration
Pulse rate	Normal to increased	Tachycardia[a]	Tachycardia or bradycardia or absent
Pulse quality	Normal	Normal to decreased	Weak, thread, impalpable
Systolic blood pressure	Normal	Normal but orthostatic	Decreased
Urine output	Normal or mildly decreased	Little or absent	No urine output for more than 8 h
% Body weight loss In infants	<5%	5–10%	>10%
In older children	<3%	3–6%	>6%

Notes:

Skin turgor and capillary refill, in addition to rate and pattern of breathing, are the best indicators for hydration status.

Skin turgor and sunken eyes are unreliable signs of dehydration in a severely malnourished child. [9]

[a]These signs are helpful in identification of children at risk for progression to shock. [7]

Table 4.2 The WHO classification of the severity of dehydration in children with diarrhea[a]

Parameters	No dehydration	Some dehydration[b]	Severe dehydration[b]
Condition	Well, alert	Restlessness, irritability	Lethargy or unconsciousness
Eyes	Normal	Sunken	Sunken
Thirst	Drinks normally, not thirsty	Drinks eagerly, thirsty	Unable to drink or drinks poorly
Skin pinch	Goes back quickly	Goes back slowly	Goes back very slowly (≥2 s)
Treatment	Plan A	Plan B	Plan C

[a]Reproduced with the permission of WHO. [10]

[b]The patient should have two or more signs.

4.4   Assessment of Nutritional Status

- Evaluation of the nutritional status of a child depends on the following parameters:
  - Detailed feeding history (see Chap. 1).
  - Clinical examination and anthropometry (growth measures) (see below).
  - Measurement of basic biochemical and hematological indices, if possible, to identify micronutrient deficiencies (outside the scope of this chapter).
- Strictly speaking, malnutrition refers to undernutrition or being overweight. However, in this chapter, the term is employed to refer specifically to undernutrition.

4.4.1 Clinical Examination to Assess Nutritional Status

1. **General condition and facial appearance**
   - A well-nourished child is active and alert, his/her cheeks are full, the buttocks are firm and rounded, the muscle tone is good, the hair is shiny, and the skin is healthy.
   - An undernourished child may appear apathic, irritable, or lethargic, and his/her face may be miserable, puffy, or "moon" shaped (kwashiorkor) or have a "monkey facies" and an aged appearance (marasmus), or the child's eyes may be sunken due to loss of periorbital fat, in addition to other signs of undernutrition (see below).

2. **Visible severe muscle wasting**
   - Undress the child. You can ask for the parent's help.
   - Loose skin folds or severe muscle wasting may be visible at the thighs, buttocks, shoulders, arms, ribs, and scapulae.
   - Look at the child from the side, noting the fat of the buttocks.
   - Inspect the child's chest and note if the outline of the child's ribs is easily seen.
   - Inspect both hips of the child and compare them with his/her chest and abdomen; they may look small.
   - In severe cases, you may see many folds of skin on the buttocks and thighs.
   - Although it eventually becomes wasted, the child's face may still look normal, even when there is severe wasting [9].

3. **Edema of both feet**
   - Inspect both of the child's feet (dorsum, in particular) to determine the presence of edema.
   - Press gently but firmly on the dorsum of each foot for 10 seconds and release, using your thumb. A residual dent in the child's foot points to the presence of pitting edema.

4. **Look for other signs that may suggest specific micronutrient deficiency, such as:**
   - **Pallor**
     - Pallor is a sign of anemia.
     - Iron deficiency is the most common micronutrient deficiency.
     - Look for pallor on the palm:
       Grasp the child's palm gently from the side to hold it open.
       Avoid stretching fingers backward because it may cause pallor by blocking the blood supply.
       Always compare the child's palm color with your palm and, if possible, with the palms of other children.
     - Paleness of the skin of the child's palm means the child has some palmar pallor. If it is very pale or so pale that it looks white, the child has severe palmar pallor [9].
   - **Signs of vitamin deficiency**, e.g., signs of rickets (suggest vitamin D deficiency), signs of scurvy (suggest vitamin C deficiency) (see below).

Table 4.3 Selected physical signs of nutritional deficiency [11, 12]

Organ/body part	Signs
Skin	Shiny and edematous skin (as in kwashiorkor) or lose and wrinkled skin (as in marasmus); dry, peeling skin with raw exposed areas; sandpaper feel of the skin; patchy excessive lightness or darkness of the skin (dyspigmentation); ecchymosis/intradermal petechia (vitamin K or C deficiencies); and jaundice
Nail	Rigid and spoon-shaped nail (koilonychia) with thin, soft nail plates
Hair	Alopecia; easily pluckable; light, brown, or reddish color; thin, sparse, and brittle hair; occasionally **flag sign** (characteristic of kwashiorkor, it refers to bands of light color alternating with normal darker hair color, representing poor nutrition and reasonable nutrition periods, respectively)
Eyes	Angular palpebritis (redness and fissuring of eyelid corners), pale conjunctiva, dryness of conjunctiva and cornea (vitamin A deficiency), corneal revascularization, keratomalacia, Bitot's spots, periorbital edema
Mouth	Cheilosis, glossitis, angular stomatitis (vitamin B2, B6, and B12 deficiencies), papillary atrophy, purplish-color tongue, and spongy bleeding gums (vitamin C deficiency)
Extremities	Widening of wrists and ankles (double malleolus), deformities (result from vitamin D, calcium, or vitamin C deficiencies), loss of deep tendon reflexes of the lower limbs (vitamin B1 and B12 deficiencies), hands and feet may be cold
Abdomen	Abdominal distention (due to poor abdominal musculature), ascites, tender hepatomegaly (due to fatty infiltration)

- **Signs of infection**, such as fever or hypothermia; hypothermia may also indicate hypoglycemia.
- Look for other signs that may suggest malnutrition (see Table 4.3).

4.4.2   Anthropometric Assessments of Nutritional Status

- Measure the child's weight and length (<2 years of age) or height (>2 years of age). In addition to these two key measurements, assess mid-upper arm circumference (MUAC), which is useful as a screening tool for malnutrition in the community. Head circumference measurement may be useful in children under 3 years of age.
- Determine weight-for-length or weight-for-height and weight-for-age, using the standard growth charts according to the child's age and sex (see Sect. 4.5).

4.4.3   Classification of Childhood Malnutrition

There are many classifications for malnutrition, for example:

- **The World Health Organization (WHO) classification of malnutrition**
  - According to the WHO, malnutrition can be graded as moderate and severe malnutrition, depending on weight-for-height (measure of wasting),

Table 4.4 Wellcome classification of malnutrition [13, 15]

	60–80% expected weight-for-age	<60% expected weight-for-age
With edema	Kwashiorkor	Marasmic kwashiorkor
Without edema	Underweight (undernutrition)	Marasmus

    height-for-age (measure of stunting), mid-upper arm circumference, and the
    presence or absence of edema [12, 13].
- – In children between 6 and 59 months of age, moderate acute malnutrition
    (MAM) is defined as a weight-for-length or weight-for-height between −2
    standard deviations (SD) and −3SD (based on the WHO Child Growth
    Standards) or a mid-arm circumference (MUAC) between 115 mm and
    125 mm, while severe acute malnutrition (SAM) is defined as the presence of
    severe wasting (weight-for-length or weight-for-height < −3SD, or mid-upper
    arm circumference (MUAC) <115 mm), or the presence of edema of both feet
    [12, 14].
- • **Wellcome classification of malnutrition**
- – The Wellcome classification of malnutrition depends on the standard weight-
    for-age and the presence or absence of edema to classify malnourished chil-
    dren into those with kwashiorkor, marasmic kwashiorkor, underweight, and
    marasmus (see Table 4.4 and Box 4.1) [15].

Box 4.1: Kwashiorkor and Marasmus

- • **Kwashiorkor** is a manifestation of severe protein and essential nutrient deficiency in the diet. It is characterized by generalized edema; hair that is thin,
  sparse, depigmented, and easily pulled out; a skin that is thickened, dry, scaly,
  smooth, and shiny over areas of edema; and a face that is puffy (the so-called
  moon face) [7, 9].
- • **Marasmus** is a manifestation of a reduction of all food intake or starvation, with
  a predominance of calorie deficiency. It is characterized by wasting, and the child
  looks to be just "skin and bones" with an "old man" appearance [9, 16].

4.5   Anthropometric Measures (Growth Parameters)

- • Growth is a vital indicator of a child's general well-being. Therefore, an accurate
  assessment of the child's growth is very important.
- • Anthropometric measures are tools for evaluating the growth and nutritional sta-
  tus of children. The most important growth parameters are:
  - – Weight
  - – Length or height
  - – Head circumference

- Mid-upper arm circumference (MUAC)
- Body mass index (BMI)
- Except in emergencies, you should routinely measure the child's weight and height or length and plot them on an appropriate growth chart in every physical examination of a child.
- Serial measurements of growth parameters are more important than a single one.
- If possible, use the same equipment at each visit.
- Compare the new measurements with the previous growth trends.
- Plot the results longitudinally on an appropriate growth chart.

4.5.1   Weight

- Use an accurate scale and calibrate it accurately to measure the child's weight.
- Infants and young children should be naked (no diaper) at the time of weight measurement.
- Older children should be weighed wearing only underwear or light clothes, without shoes or socks.
- Plot the measured weight on an appropriate growth chart.

Notes 4.1

- You can determine a child's expected weight in kilograms, based on his/her age, using the following formulas:
  - Child's weight at 3–12 months = (age in months + 9)/2
  - Child's weight at 1–6 years = 2(age in years) + 8
  - Child's weight at 7–12 years = (7 × age in years – 5)/2
- If the child's age and birth weight are known, you can simply estimate his/her current weight in kilograms by using the following formulas:
  - Weight at 4–5 months = birth weight × 2
  - Weight at 1 year = birth weight × 3
  - Weight at 2 years = birth weight × 4
  - Weight at 7 years = birth weight × 7
  - Weight at 10 years = birth weight × 10

4.5.2   Length or Height

- Measurement of infant's length
  - Use an infantometer to measure the supine length of children aged less than 2 years or of those with a handicap.
  - Ask an assistant (the child's parent, if possible) to hold the child's head against the headboard.
  - Move the footboard firmly up against the child's heels, and, before taking the reading of length, make sure that his/her feet are at 90° and the legs are straight (see Fig. 4.1).

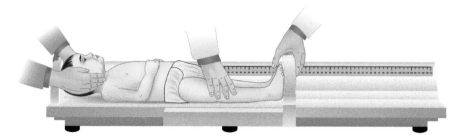

Fig. 4.1 Method of measurement of an infant's length by infantometer

- Measurement of the child's height
  - Use a stadiometer to measure the standing height of children <u>older than 2 years of age</u>.
  - The child should stand erect with the feet bare and the scapulae, buttocks, and heels all touching the backboard; the knees should be straight.
  - A gentle, upward traction should be applied to the mastoid process to extend the neck, and make sure the child's eyes are in the same plane with the external auditory meatus (see Fig. 4.2).
  - Plot the measured length or height on an appropriate growth chart.

Notes 4.2

- There is a diurnal variation in the height of children (up to 2 cm). Therefore, to get an accurate determination of the height velocity, it is preferable to take the measure of the child's height at the same time of the day at each visit—if possible, in the afternoon [17].

Notes 4.3

- The length or height of children can be roughly estimated according to their age:

Age	Expected length or height
At birth	50 cm
6 months	66 cm
1 year	75 cm
2 years	89 cm
3 years	95 cm
4½ years	105 cm
5–10 years	105 cm, plus 5–6 cm for each year

- In children aged 2–12 years, height can also be estimated by using the following formula: child's height in centimeters = 6(age in years) + 77

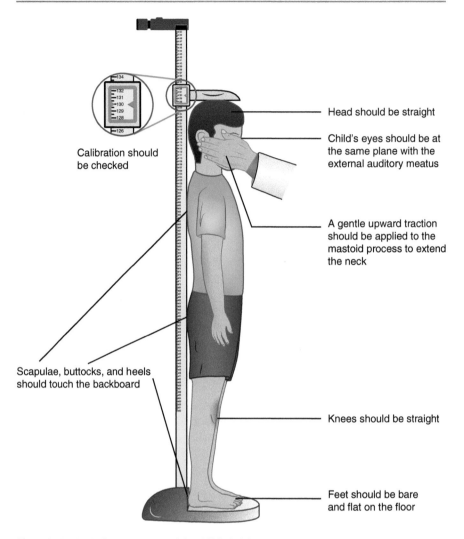

Fig. 4.2 Method of measurement of the child's height

4.5.3   Head Circumference

- Head circumference represents the growth of the child's brain.
- Use a flexible, but non-stretchable, tape to measure the maximum occipitofrontal circumference in <u>children under 36 months</u>.
- The landmarks for the measurement are the superior orbital ridge (just above the eyes), at the front, and the external occipital protuberance, at the back (see Fig. 4.3).
- Repeat the measurement three times and take the largest diameter.
- Plot the measured head circumference on an appropriate growth chart.

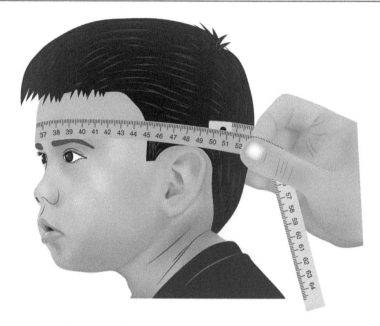

Fig. 4.3 Method of head circumference measurement

Clinical Tips 4.3

- If the measured circumference of the child's head is significantly greater or lower than normal, take the measurements of each of the parents' heads, especially the father, and see whether these measurements fit on the chart or not. Familial large or small head is not uncommon [1].

Notes 4.4

- Head circumference increases with age as follows:
  - 2 cm per month in the first 3 months of age
  - 1 cm per month from 3 to 6 months of age
  - 0.5 cm per month from 6 months to 1 year of age
- The average head circumference can be calculated simply according to the child's age, as follows [1, 13]:

Age	Head circumference in centimeters
At birth	35 cm
3 months	41 cm
6 months	44 cm
1 year	46 cm
2 years	48 cm
5 years	50 cm
15 years	55 cm

4.5.4   Mid-Upper Arm Circumference (MUAC)

Use a non-stretchable tape to measure the mid-upper arm circumference (MUAC) at the midpoint between the tip of the shoulder (the acromion) and the tip of the elbow (the olecranon process) (see Fig. 4.4).

> **Notes 4.5**
>
> - Mid-upper arm circumference (MUAC) is a useful screening tool to detect malnutrition in the community in the situations where resources are limited or when the child's weight is misleading, as in cases of cancer, edema, or liver diseases [15].
> - MUAC at birth is 10 cm, while it is relatively constant in children between 6 months and 5 years, ranging from 16 to 17 cm. Measurements of >13.5 cm are considered normal [13].

4.5.5   Body Mass Index (BMI)

- Body mass index is a useful index of thinness, overweight, and obesity in children.
- It can be calculated by dividing the child's weight (in kilograms) by the square of the height (in meters).
- Normal BMI is 18.5–25 kg/m².

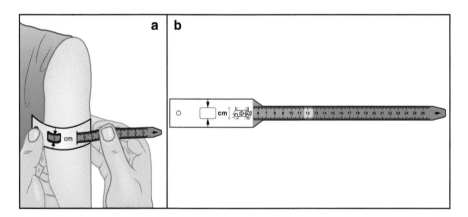

Fig. 4.4 (**a**) Method of measuring the mid-upper arm circumference (MUAC). (**b**) Mid-upper arm circumference (MUAC) measuring tape. A measurement in the green zone (from 12.5 cm) means the child is well nourished; a measurement in the yellow zone (11.5–12.5 cm) indicates that the child is at risk of acute malnutrition; a measurement in the red zone (0–11.5 cm) signifies that the child is acutely malnourished. If this tape is not available, you can use any flexible, non-stretchable tape instead

4.5.6 Growth Charts

- Growth charts are very important tools for assessing the growth of a child.
- Health professionals can monitor the growth and nutritional status of a child by measuring the child's anthropometric parameters and plotting the measurements on an appropriate growth chart—e.g., the WHO Child Growth Standards, which are recommended in many countries (see Fig. 4.5). This is helpful in comparing the child's growth measurements with the measurements of normal children of the same age and sex.
- The calculations of weight-for-age, weight-for-height, and height-for-age are very important in the assessment of the child's growth and nutritional status (see Box 4.2).
- The choice of an appropriate growth chart depends mainly on the child's age (in months), sex, and the measured parameters.
- The measurement of the child should be marked on the chart with a dot (not a cross or a circle).

Clinical Tips 4.4

- When the evaluated child's growth does not follow a normal pattern, consider factors that may influence the growth, such as parental stature, birth weight, gestational age, nutrition, type of feeding (breast or formula), environment, or chronic illness.

4.6 Vital Signs

There are four main vital signs: pulse rate (heart rate), respiratory rate, temperature, and blood pressure. These signs vary steadily with the child's age and activity (see Table 4.5) [16, 23].

Box 4.2: Important Growth Indicators

- **Weight-for-age** is the most widely used index for evaluation of nutritional status, though it does not differentiate wasting from stunting.
- **Weight-for-height** (or weight-for-length, for children under 2 years old) is a partially age-independent index. Low values indicate wasting and point to acute malnutrition, while high values may indicate overweight status. Currently, this parameter should be the preferred choice over the simple weight and/or height in isolation [19].
- **Height-for-age** (or length-for-age, for children under 2 years old) detects stunting and points to chronic malnutrition.

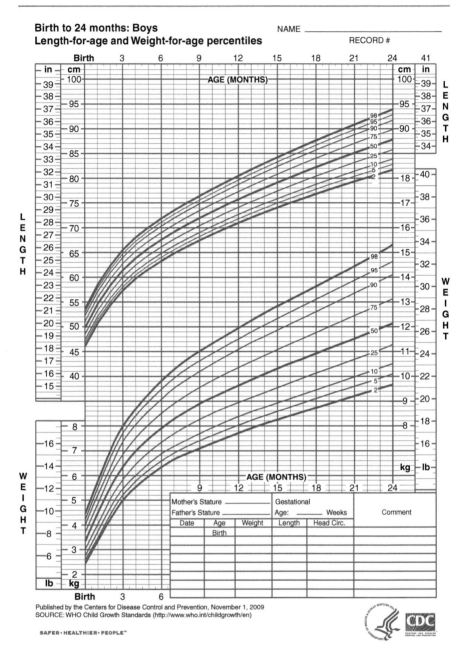

Fig. 4.5 Sample growth chart. Percentile standards for length-for-age and weight-for-age in boys, birth to age 24 months (Centers for Disease Control and Prevention. November 1, 2009. Source: WHO Child Growth Standards—http://www.who.int/childgrowth/standards/en/) [18]

Table 4.5 Normal ranges of the resting pulse rate, respiratory rate, and systolic blood pressure, according to the child's age [20–22]

Age	Pulse rate (beats/min)	Respiratory rate (breaths/min)	Systolic blood pressure (mmHg)
Birth	100–160	30–60	50–70
1–2 years	100–150	25–35	80–95
2–5 years	95–140	20–30	80–100
5–12 years	80–120	14–22	90–110
>12 years	60–100	12–18	100–120

4.6.1 Pulse Rate (Heart Rate)

- Assess heart rate and rhythm by direct auscultation of the heart or by palpation of the peripheral arterial pulses (the brachial artery in infants and radial artery in older children). By palpation of the pulse, you can assess the pulse rate, rhythm, character, as well as volume [23] (see Sect. 4.9).
- Significant tachycardia should be considered when the heart rate is >200 beats/min in newborns, >150 beats/min in infants, and > 120 beats/min in older children [24].

4.6.2 Respiratory Rate

- To measure the respiratory rate, the child should be quiet or asleep.
- Observe chest movements (in older children) or abdominal movements (in infants and young children), and count the number of respirations over 1 min (as infants have irregular respirations).
- In older children, pretend to be measuring the child's radial pulse while observing the respiration.

Notes 4.6

- Rapid breathing above the normal range for the child's age is termed **tachypnea**, and it may occur as a response to exercise, fear, fever, or pain; it may also be a sign of conditions such as pneumonia, sepsis, aspiration, pneumothorax, pulmonary embolism, or heart failure.
- A slow respiratory rate (i.e., below the normal range of respiration for the child's age) is termed as **bradypnea**, and it may be non-pathological or may occur as a response to CNS depressants or other conditions, such as hydrocephalus or a CNS tumor [23].

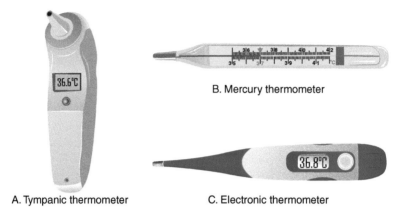

A. Tympanic thermometer   C. Electronic thermometer

B. Mercury thermometer

Fig. 4.6 Different types of thermometers

4.6.3   Temperature

- Use a sterile, accurate, electronic, mercury, or tympanic infrared thermometer to measure the child's temperature (see Fig. 4.6).
- Body temperature measurements are varied at various body sites of measurement (oral, axillary, rectal, or tympanic) (see Table 4.6) [20].

Notes 4.7

- There is a normal variation of about 1 °C in the body temperature with time of day. The lowest temperature occurs in early morning (2–6 a.m.), while the highest occurs in early evening (5–7 p.m.) [23, 27].

Table 4.6 Normal ranges and means of the body temperature at various body sites [25, 26]

Site of measurement	Normal range (°C)	Normal mean (°C)[a]
Oral	35.5–37.5	36.6
Axillary	34.7–37.3	36.4
Rectal	36.6–37.9	37.0
Tympanic	35.7–37.5	36.6

[a]An increment of 1 °C or more above these mean values is considered a fever.

4.6.3.1 General Tips for Temperature Measurement

- Clean the thermometer before and after each measurement.
- Shake down a mercury thermometer to 35° or below before each use.

Oral Thermometry

- Measuring of oral temperature is preferred <u>for children older than 5 years of age who can cooperate</u>.
- Drinking hot or cold liquids and breathing through the mouth can alter the reading of the temperature [28].

Method of Measurement

1. Insert the tip of a sterile thermometer under the child's tongue.
2. Instruct the child to close his/her mouth and breathe through the nose.
3. Wait for 2–3 min. (A digital thermometer usually takes about 10 s to measure the temperature.)
4. Remove the thermometer and read the temperature.

Axillary Thermometry

- Axillary thermometry has less sensitivity in the detection of fever than other methods.
- It is more accurate in neonates than in older infants and children [4].

Method of Measurement

1. Place the tip of the thermometer deeply into the armpit, and hold the upper arm tightly against the side for 3–5 min [13, 27].
2. Then remove the thermometer and read the temperature.

Rectal Thermometry

- Rectal thermometry is preferred in <u>infants</u> and <u>young children under 4 years of age</u>.
- It is the most useful method to measure a baby's core temperature [23].

Method of Measurement

1. Use an appropriate lubricant (e.g., Vaseline) to lubricate the tip of the thermometer.
2. Place the baby prone and gently separate his/her buttocks.
3. Insert the thermometer, without force, about 2–3 cm into the rectum, and hold it in place for at least 2 min.
4. Then remove the thermometer from the rectum and read the temperature.

Infrared Tympanic Membrane Thermometry
- Infrared tympanic membrane thermometry is an easy, safe, fast, and practical method to take a child's temperature, with no risk of cross-infection, and it can accurately reflect the core body temperature [27].

Method of Measurement

1. Retract the pinna gently and insert the disposable probe into the external auditory canal. Then watch for the digital readout (after about 2–3 s).
2. Then remove the tympanic thermometer and read the temperature.
3. Repeat the measurement twice and record the higher one.

4.6.4 Blood Pressure

- As part of a physical examination, blood pressure should be measured in <u>any child aged 3 years or older</u> and <u>in younger children with a history or examination that may suggest abnormal blood pressure</u>.
- Normal blood pressure values vary, depending on the child's age, sex, and height.

4.6.4.1 Method of Measurement (See Fig. 4.7)

1. Blood pressure measurement should be taken in a quiet room.
2. Explain the procedure to the child and his/her parents.
3. The child should be relaxed and rested, in either a sitting or supine position.
4. Blood pressure should be recorded in the right arm.
5. Calculate the length of the child's arm by measuring the distance between the olecranon of the elbow and the acromion process.
6. Use an accurate sphygmomanometer, with a proper cuff size. The rubber bag must have an appropriate width that covers two-thirds of the child's arm; it must also have a suitable length that covers at least three-fourths of the upper arm circumference. A narrow cuff yields falsely high-pressure readings, while a too-wide cuff underestimates the blood pressure [29].
7. Apply the cuff to the child's upper arm and make sure that it fits firmly.
8. Localize the brachial artery in the antecubital fossa medial to the bicep tendon.
9. Ensure that the midpoint of the rubber bag (which is inside the cuff) is above the brachial artery.
10. The child's arm (antecubital fossa) must be at the level of the child's heart.
11. Palpate the brachial or radial pulse and inflate the cuff until disappearance of the pulse.
12. Deflate the cuff and note at which pressure the pulse reappears. This is the palpatory systolic pressure.
13. After 15 s, reinflate the cuff to about 30 mmHg more than the measured palpatory systolic pressure.

14. Place the diaphragm of the stethoscope over the brachial artery pulse, and make sure that it is not touching the cuff or the tubes.
15. Deflate the cuff of the sphygmomanometer gradually, at a rate of about 2–3 mmHg/s, and listen carefully to the appearance of the first Korotkoff sounds. These indicate systolic blood pressure. The sounds start out louder and then become muffled and disappear.
16. The muffling or disappearance of these sounds indicates the diastolic blood pressure.
17. Measure the blood pressure twice, since the child will become more relaxed.
18. The pulse rate should be measured with each measurement of blood pressure. A high pulse rate may indicate anxiety, elevating the blood pressure.
19. If the child has a history of postural hypotension, you must measure the standing blood pressure.
20. Plot the reading of the blood pressure on a special chart for blood pressure.
21. At the end of the procedure, tell the parent or the child (if old enough) the blood pressure reading, and discuss its significance, and then thank the child and the parents.

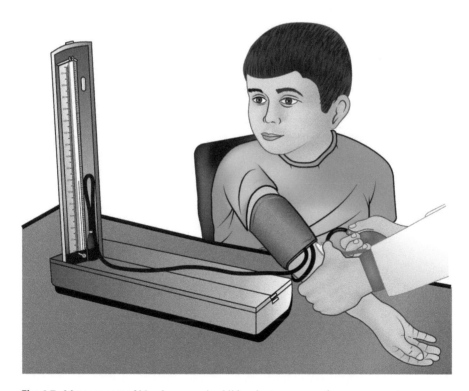

Fig. 4.7 Measurement of blood pressure in children by a mercury sphygmomanometer

Notes 4.8

- In infants, blood pressure is measured by ultrasound (Doppler) devices, as it may be difficult to obtain by the above-described method [29].
- A high blood pressure reading requires measurement of the blood pressure in the other hand and at least one leg.
- Blood pressure can be measured in the leg with the child in a prone position. The rubber bag should be wide enough to cover two-thirds of the thigh length and long enough to cover three-fourths of the thigh circumference. Place the stethoscope on the popliteal artery and repeat the same procedure.
- Normally, the pressure recorded in the lower extremities is higher than that measured in the upper extremities by about 10 mmHg [24].

4.7   Examination of the Skin, Hair, and Nails

- Examination of the skin requires good light. Daylight is best; if unavailable, the next-best choice is fluorescent lighting.
- Use of a magnifying lens is helpful for recognition of details.
- With adequate exposure, examine the entire skin surface, even when the history suggests a localized lesion.

Examination Station 4.1: Examination of the Skin, Hair, and Nails

1. **Skin Examination**
   - **Inspection**
     - Color
     - Uniformity
     - Hygiene
     - Odors
     - Abnormalities
       Any skin lesions. If there is a lesion, note its morphology, configuration, location, distribution, color, border, and the presence of pus or exudate
       Abnormal pigmentation and birthmarks
       Bleeding: petechiae, purpura, ecchymosis, and hematoma
   - **Palpation**
     - Texture (character)
     - Moisture
     - Turgor (skin tension or elasticity)

Continued on the next page

- Temperature
- Edema
2. **Hair Examination**
   - **Inspection**
     - Color
     - Cleanliness
     - Quantity
     - Distribution
     - Abnormalities (e.g., hair loss, excessive hair, seborrhea, or nits)
   - **Palpation**
     - Texture
3. **Nails Examination**
   - **Inspection**
     - Shape and contour
     - Length
     - Color and any abnormal pigmentation
     - Symmetry
     - Cleanliness
     - Nail-base angle
     - Proximal and lateral nail folds
     - Abnormalities
   - **Palpation**
     - Palpate the nail plate for the following: texture, firmness, thickness, and uniformity
     - Palpate the proximal and lateral nail folds for tenderness

4.7.1   Skin Examination

1. **Inspection**

   Inspect the skin color. Check for jaundice, pallor, cyanosis, or plethora. Note the uniformity of the skin, hygiene, and any abnormal odors. Also, look for any:

   (a) Skin lesion: Inspect and palpate the lesion to determine the following:
   - **Morphology** (the type of the lesion)
     - Primary skin lesions: result from the disease itself and are unmodified by external factors [30]
       Macule: flat discoloration, <1 cm in diameter, e.g., freckles
       Patch: flat discoloration, >1 cm in diameter, e.g., port wine stains
       Papule: elevated, superficial, <1 cm in diameter, e.g., molluscum contagiosum
       Plaque: elevated, superficial, >1 cm in diameter, e.g., psoriasis
       Nodule: elevated with a deeper component, >1 cm in diameter, e.g., erythema nodosum

Pustule: collection of pus, <1 cm in diameter, e.g., folliculitis

Vesicle: collection of clear fluid, <1 cm in diameter, e.g., herpes simplex

Bulla: collection of clear fluid, >1 cm in diameter, e.g., bullous impetigo

Wheal: transient, elevated, flat-topped lesion, occurs due to dermal edema, e.g., urticaria

– Secondary skin lesions: evolve from primary lesions or caused by external factors, such as scratching or trauma

Scale: flakes of dead epidermal cells (e.g., seborrheic dermatitis)

Crust: a collection of cellular debris, dried serum, blood, or pus (e.g., impetigo)

Scar: an abnormal formation of fibrous tissue after wound healing (e.g., scar of acne)

Fissure: a linear slit in the skin (e.g., angular cheilitis)

Atrophy: a depression in the skin as a result of thinning of the epidermis, dermis, or subcutis (e.g., lichen sclerosis)

Lichenifcation: a thickening of the epidermis with accentuation of normal skin markings (e.g., chronic eczema)

Erosion: a complete or partial focal loss of epidermis, heals without scar (e.g., impetigo)

Excoriation: an erosion occurring due to an exogenous injury (e.g., atopic dermatitis)

Ulcer: a full-thickness focal loss of epidermis with loss of at least part of dermis, or even subcutis, healed with a scar (e.g., pressure ulcers)

• **Configuration** (the shape or outline of a single skin lesion or the arrangement of lesions with each other), for example:
  – Dermatomal (e.g., herpes zoster)
  – Clustered (e.g., herpes simplex)
  – Linear (e.g., linear epidermal nevi)
  – Target or iris (e.g., erythema multiforme)
  – Reticular (e.g., erythema infectiosum)
  – Annular (e.g., tinea corporis)
  – Nummular (e.g., nummular eczema)
• **Location and distribution**
  – Localized (e.g., impetigo) or generalized (e.g., urticaria)
  – Region of the body: in the sun-exposed area (e.g., photodermatitis, sunburn); on the face, shoulder, and back (e.g., acne); and on the extensors aspect of the extremities (e.g., psoriasis)
  – Single or multiple lesions
  – Symmetrical or asymmetrical distribution
• **Color of the lesion**
  – Red (e.g., port-wine stains)
  – Yellow (e.g., xanthomas)
  – Blue (e.g., deep dermal nevi)
  – Black (e.g., melanoma)
• **Borders:** Regular or irregular, well-demarcated or blurred
• **Pus or exudate:** Note color, odor, amount, and consistency.

(b) Abnormal pigmentations and birthmarks (see Chap. 3).
(c) Bleeding into the skin or mucosa, which does not blanch on pressure:
  • Petechiae: non-blanching, red-purple, fine spots, <1 mm in diameter
  • Purpura: non-blanching, red-purple spots, 2–10 mm in diameter
    – Palpable (e.g., meningococcal septicemia and Henoch–Schönlein purpura)
    – Non-palpable (e.g., thrombocytopenia)
  • Ecchymosis: a non-blanching, large bruise
  • Hematoma: a bleeding into the skin large enough to produce a tender elevation

2. **Palpation**

After the inspection, palpate the skin to determine the following:
  (a) **Texture** (the character of the skin surface): Normally, the skin has an even, soft, and smooth texture.
  (b) **Moisture**: Wetness and oiliness of the skin
  (c) **Turgor** (normal fullness state; it reflects skin tension or elasticity): Assess the skin turgor by pinching a fold of the skin on the sternal area (or on the abdomen near the umbilicus), and gently twist it with your fingertips and release. Normally, it lifts easily and returns back to its resting position immediately. Skin turgor is reduced or lost in dehydration and marasmus [5].
  (d) **Temperature**: Palpate for the temperature with the dorsum of your hand, comparing side by side. The temperature may reflect the blood flow through the dermis. Normal skin is warm.
  (e) **Edema**: Pitting or non-pitting

Clinical Tips 4.5

• If there is a skin lesion, in addition to palpation for its texture, it is important to ascertain whether it is blanchable (i.e., disappears with pressure, occurs due to vasodilatation) or non-blanchable (i.e., occurs due to extravasation of red blood cells into the tissue, e.g., purpura).

4.7.2 Hair Examination

• **Inspection**
• Inspect the scalp, eyebrows, eyelashes, axillary, and body hair, looking for the color, cleanliness, distribution, and quantity, and note any abnormalities, such as:
  – Hair loss: localized or diffuse
  – Excessive hair: hypertrichosis or hirsutism
  – Others: seborrhea, lice, nits, or dandruff, and note any associated skin conditions
• **Palpation**
  – Palpate scalp hair for texture, noting whether it has fine, medium, or coarse texture (see Key Points 4.1).

Key Points 4.1

- Scalp hair is straight or curly, coarse or fine, smooth, shiny, and resilient, while dry and brittle hair is abnormal.
- Dry, coarse hair may occur in hypothyroidism, while fine, thin hair may be a sign of homocystinuria.
- When there is a localized hair loss, it is very important to inspect the scalp for accompanied scarring or inflammation.
- The hair of infants tends to fall out by the third month of life and is replaced by hair that may differ markedly in color, distribution, and texture.

4.7.3   Nails Examination

- **Inspection**
  Inspect the nails, looking for:
  - Shape and contour.
  - Color: Normal nail-bed color should be a variation of pink.
  - Length, symmetry, and configuration.
  - Cleanliness.
  - Nail-base angle: Normally this measures 160°. In case of clubbing of the finger, it may exceed 180° (see Fig. 4.8 and Box 4.3).

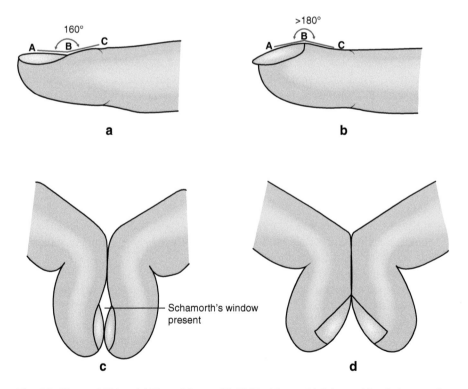

Fig. 4.8   Finger clubbing. (**a**) Normal finger. (**b**) Clubbed finger. (**c**) Schamroth's window test for a normal finger. (**d**) Schamroth's window test for a clubbed finger

- The proximal and lateral nail folds: Inspect the proximal and lateral nail folds, noting the following: redness, discharge, swelling, and any lesions, such as warts.
- Abnormalities, e.g., absent nail, platonychia (flat nails with loss of normal convexity), koilonychia (spoon-shaped nails), leukonychia (due to chronic states of hypoalbuminemia, e.g., nephrotic syndrome, protein-losing enteropathy), splinter hemorrhage (may suggest trauma, vasculitis, nail psoriasis, or endocarditis), and pitted nails (suggests psoriasis, eczema, or alopecia areata).

- **Palpation**
  - Palpate the nail plate for the following: texture, firmness, thickness, and uniformity, noting its adherence to the nail bed by gently squeezing the nail plate with your thumb and index finger.
  - Palpate the proximal and lateral nail folds for tenderness.

Key Points 4.2

- Changes in nail color may indicate pathology (e.g., green–black discoloration is suggestive of pseudomonas infection; periungual brown–black discoloration may suggest melanoma, while a completely blue nail suggests diseases that may cause cyanosis, such as cyanotic congenital heart disease).
- The normal nail plate should be smooth and hard, with a uniform thickness.
- The complete absence of a nail may suggest congenital syndromes (e.g., nail–patella syndrome).

Box 4.3: Finger Clubbing

- A clubbed finger is characterized by swelling of the soft tissue of the terminal phalanges and obliteration of the normal angle between the nail plate and the proximal nail fold.
- It starts as softening and increased boggy fluctuation of the nail bed, followed by loss of the normal angle between the nail plate and the proximal nail fold, then the increment in thickness and curvature of the nail plate, and finally the fingers may have a drumstic appearance. Finger clubbing occurs due to many causes listed in Table 4.7.
- A simple way to measure the nail-base angle is the Schamroth's technique, having the child place together the dorsal surface of the nail of the index fingers or thumbs of both hands; disappearance of the diamond-shaped window indicates finger clubbing (see Fig. 4.8c, d).

Table 4.7 Causes of clubbing of fingers and toes [3, 4]

Familial causes (5–10%)

Acquired causes

Respiratory diseases	Cardiovascular diseases	Gastrointestinal diseases	Miscellaneous
• Chronic suppurative lung disease – Bronchiectasis – Lung abscess – Cystic fibrosis – Empyema • Progressive pulmonary tuberculosis • Pulmonary fibrosis • Lung cancer	• Cyanotic congenital heart disease • Infective endocarditis • Arteriovenous shunts and aneurysms	• Inflammatory bowel disease (Crohn's disease and ulcerative colitis) • Celiac disease • Tropical sprue • Multiple polyposis • Liver cirrhosis • Chronic active hepatitis	• Thyrotoxicosis (thyroid acropathy) • Hodgkin lymphoma • Syringomyelia

4.8   Examination of the Head, Face, and Neck

Examination Station 4.2: Examination of the Head, Face, and Neck

1. **Head Examination**
   - Inspection: shape and abnormalities
   - Palpation: fontanels, bones, and sutures
   - Auscultation: over the vertex, temple, and eyeball for harsh and loud bruit
   - Transillumination: done in a dark room to detect severe hydrocephalus, chronic subdural hematoma, effusion, and hydranencephaly
   - Measurements: head circumference
2. **Face Examination**
   - Dysmorphic features
   - Eyes examination
     - External inspection: shape, symmetry, orientation, alignment, abnormalities
     - Eye function: reflexes, eye movements, vision, color vision
     - Fundoscopy
   - Ear examination
     - Inspection: shape, position, patency
     - Palpation: swelling and tenderness
     - Hearing assessment
     - Otoscopy

Continued on the next page

- Nose examination
  - Inspection: shape, size, and condition
  - Evaluation for patency of nostrils
  - Palpation of sinuses for tenderness
- Mouth and throat examination
  - Inspection: the lips, tongue, teeth, buccal mucosa, gum, tonsils, and palate
  - Palpation: the lips and hard palate

3. **Neck Examination**
   - Inspection: symmetry, contour, and abnormalities (e.g., shortness, torticollis, masses, or scar)
   - Range of movement: limitation in neck movement or pain
   - Palpation: trachea, lymph nodes, and any masses or tenderness

4.8.1 Head Examination

- **Inspection**
  - Note the shape of child's head (see Box 4.4).
  - Look for frontal bossing (prominence of forehead occurs in rickets, untreated thalassemia, congenital syphilis, polysaccharidosis, and mucopolysaccharidosis), shiny skin, shunt, or dilated veins.

Box 4.4: Important Terms

- **Macrocephaly** (large head) is defined as a baby's head circumference of more than two standard deviations (SD) above the mean for his/her age and sex. It may be familial (in 50% of cases) or may indicate certain pathologies (e.g., hydrocephalus) [31, 32].
- **Microcephaly** (very small head) is defined as a baby's head circumference more than three standard deviations (SD) below the mean for his/her age and sex. It may be a primary (e.g., familial, trisomy 21) or a secondary result from severe brain damage (e.g., congenital infections or maternal drug use) [31–33].
- **Plagiocephaly** (parallelogram head): Head asymmetry with flattening of one side, due to pressure on that side, as the healthy infant is lying with his/her head persistently on one side. Plagiocephaly usually improves with age.
- **Brachycephaly** (flat head): Decrement in the anteroposterior (AP) diameter of the head.
- **Scaphocephaly** (boat-shaped head): Increased anteroposterior (AP) diameter because of premature closure of the sagittal suture.

- **Palpation**
  - With the child in a sitting position or being held upright, palpate the anterior and posterior fontanels with your fingers to determine their size and tension and whether they are bulging (e.g., crying, meningitis, or hydrocephalus), sunken (e.g., dehydration), or flat. In a healthy, quiet infant, the anterior fontanel is very slightly depressed and may be pulsatile. Delayed closure of the fontanels may be seen in hydrocephalus, rickets, scurvy, Down syndrome, hypothyroidism, mucopolysaccharidoses, achondroplasia, etc.
  - Palpate the bones of the skull and the cranial sutures, looking for any abnormalities, such as:
    Craniosynostosis: A premature fusion of the cranial sutures occurs as an isolated condition or as part of a syndrome. Ossification of the sutures normally occurs <u>by 6 months of age</u>.
    Sutural diastasis (abnormal separation of the sutures), e.g., hydrocephalus.
    Craniotabes: The skull bones are soft and can be indented, similar to a ping-pong ball. Although it may be normal, it may suggest rickets, congenital syphilis, or osteogenesis imperfect.

Clinical Tips 4.6

- After the sutures have closed, raised intracranial pressure may be detected by elicitation of the cracked pot sound through percussion over child's skull with a finger. This is also known as the crack-pot sign or Macewen's sign. It does not always indicate hydrocephalus.

- **Auscultation**
  - Auscultate over the vertex, temple, and eyeball, listening for the presence of a harsh and loud bruit, which may suggest arteriovenous malformation or transmission of abnormal sounds from the heart or great vessels. Soft bruits or flow noises may be a normal finding in children.
- **Transillumination**
  - Transillumination of the head is not a part of the routine physical examination, but it can be useful within <u>the first year of life</u> when the child has a large asymmetric head with wide sutures. It can be examined in a dark room by applying a full-sized flashlight closely at the scalp and moving it over the entire head. A visible 1–2 cm rim of light around the margin of the flashlight is a normal finding. Increased transillumination (more than 2 cm in the frontal and 1 cm in the occipital region) can be seen in severe hydrocephalus, chronic subdural hematoma, or effusion and hydranencephaly.
- **Measurements**
  - Measure the head circumference using a non-stretchable tape (see Sect. 4.5.3).

4.8.2   Face Examination

- Note any facial asymmetry or dysmorphic features.
- Look at the jaw size, excluding abnormalities such as micrognathia (an underdeveloped jaw), which can be seen in many syndromes (e.g., Pierre Robin syndrome).

Eyes Examination
- **External inspection**
  - Note the eyes' shape, size, and orientation, and examine for photophobia.
  - Inspect the eyebrow, eyelids, eyelashes, and the eyeballs, noting any gross abnormalities, such as sunken eyes, setting-sun eye phenomenon (hydrocephalus or intracranial tumor), exophthalmos, strabismus, epicanthic folds (familial or seen in Down syndrome), hyper- or hypotelorism, puffy eyelids, ptosis, excess tearing, or any other eye abnormalities.
  - Retract the lower eyelids gently, inspecting the sclerae for jaundice or discoloration.
  - Look at the conjunctivae for any redness, subconjunctival hemorrhages, swelling, discharge (as in Gonorrhea), or pallor.
  - Examine the cornea and irises for any abnormalities, e.g., corneal opacities, megalocornea (in glaucoma).
  - Note the pupils' shape and size, as well as reaction to light.
  - See whether the child is able to fixate, and note the presence of nystagmus.
  - Examine for eye alignment:
    Note the symmetry of corneal light reflex (see Fig. 4.9).
    Perform the cover–uncover test to identify strabismus (see Fig. 4.10). This test should be performed while the child is looking at interesting near (33 cm) and distant (6 m) objects. A valid test requires good eye movement and vision. Cover one eye and watch the other. When the fixing eye is covered, the squinting eye moves rapidly to fix on the object. If you remove the cover, the squinting eye moves away again. Repeat the same procedure on the other eye.
- **Assess eye function**
  - Examine the direct and consensual pupillary reactions to light and the accommodation reflex, noting the size and symmetry of the pupils.
  - Eye movements (see Sect. 4.14.3.2).
  - Visual field (see Sect. 4.14.3.2).
  - Assess visual acuity by different methods, according to the child's age (see Sect. 4.14.3.2).
  - Conduct a color vision test using Ishihara color plates or Hardy Rand Littler.
- **Fundoscopy**
  - Test for the red reflexes of both eyes. If it is absent or partly obscured (suggests a cataract or a retinoblastoma), perform formal fundoscopy at the end of the examination (see Sect. 4.14.3.2).

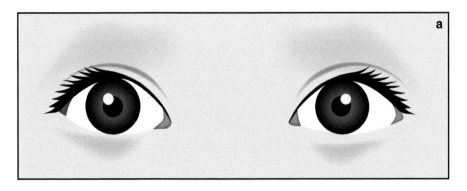

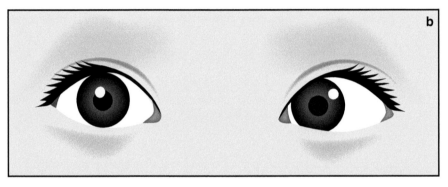

Fig. 4.9 Corneal light reflex test. Note the position of light reflection in the two eyes. (**a**) Symmetrical corneal light reflex (normal eyes). (**b**) Asymmetrical corneal light reflex (left convergent squint)

Ear Examination
- Ask the parent to hold his/her child in the proper position (see Fig. 4.11).
- Inspect the shape, position, and size of the ears, and look for any abnormalities, like ear absence, nondevelopment of the auricle, and preauricular tags. Auricular malformations may be associated with renal anomalies.
- Normally, if a continuous horizontal imaginary line is drawn from the outer canthus to the ear, it divides the ear into the upper one-third and lower two-thirds. Passage of this line above the top of the pinna indicates low-set ears, which occur in Down syndrome, Turner syndrome, and mucopolysaccharidoses.
- Note the external auditory meatus to determine whether it looks normal or not, and look for any ear discharge.
- Palpate the external ear for any swelling or tenderness.
- Percuss the mastoid bone for tenderness.
- Test for hearing by observing the child's responses to sound. Normally, he/she will turn his/her head toward the direction of the sound.
- Perform an otoscopic examination (see Box 4.5).

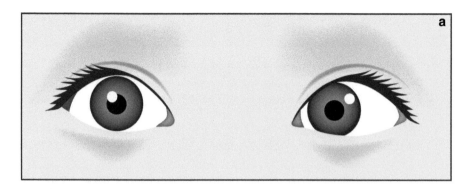

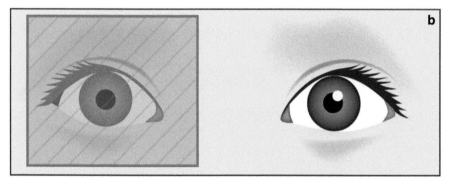

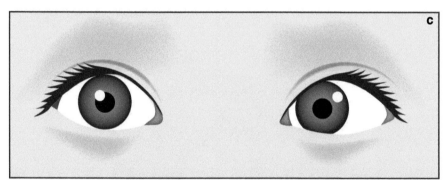

Fig. 4.10 The cover–uncover test. (**a**) Left convergent squint. Note the asymmetrical corneal light reflex. (**b**) Covering of the fixing eye results in a rapid movement of the squinting eye to fix on the object. (**c**) If you remove the cover, the squinting eye moves away again

Nose Examination

- Note the shape and size of the nose, and inspect the nostrils, nasal mucosa, and septum, looking for any abnormalities (such as nasal flaring, nasal discharge, bleeding, swelling, polyp, or foreign body).
- Evaluate the patency of the nostrils: close one nostril with your figure, and note whether the child breathes easily, verifying the patency of the other nostril.
- Palpate sinuses for tenderness.

Box 4.5: Otoscopy

- The child must be positioned properly (see Fig. 4.11).
- When the child has pain in one ear, examine the other ear first.
- The largest speculum that can fit comfortably into the child's meatus should be selected.
- The pinna must be gently pulled backward and downward (in infants and toddlers), or backward and upward (in older children), to make the external auditory canal straight.
- The otoscope should be held comfortably, and the ulnar border of your hand should be gently rested against the child's cheek.
- The otoscope should be gently inserted up to 5 mm (in infants) or 1 cm (in older children), and the angle should be adjusted until visualization of the tympanic membrane is possible.
- Normally, the tympanic membrane appears pearly gray and translucent with a cone of light reflex on it. The absence of the cone of light reflex suggests inflammation.
- Look for any signs of ear infection (e.g., redness, bulging), and note any wax, foreign body, or tympanic membrane perforation.

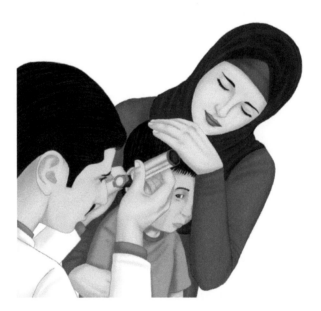

Fig. 4.11 Method of holding a child's head for ear examination. The child's head is immobilized and the hands are kept out of the way. © Anwar Qais Saadoon

Mouth and Throat Examination

- Ask the parent to hold the child properly (see Fig. 4.12).
- With the child's mouth closed, inspect and palpate the lips, noting their color, symmetry, and condition, as well as any abnormalities (such as pallor, bluish-purple discoloration, cleft lips, fissures, or dryness).
- Inspect the mouth, using a tongue depressor and a penlight, looking at the following:
  - **Teeth:** Color, number, arrangement, condition, and occlusion, noting any dental caries and loose or missing teeth
  - **Buccal mucosa:** Color and condition, looking for any abnormalities (e.g., aphthous ulcers)
  - **Gum:** Color and condition, noting any gum bleeding or hypertrophy
  - **Tongue:** Size, symmetry, color, and dorsum surface, noting any large tongue (macroglossia), fissuring of the tongue (e.g., scrotal tongue in Down syndrome), tongue tie, strawberry tongue (a swollen and bumpy tongue with large, red papillae can be seen with Kawasaki disease or scarlet fever), ulcers, or oral thrush (whitish discoloration of the tongue with an erythematous raw base, which is difficult to wipe away with the tongue depressor)
  - **Tonsils:** Size, looking for any enlarged tonsils and noting any other abnormalities (e.g., erythema, edema, and exudate).
  - **Palate:** Inspect and palpate the hard palate to exclude any abnormalities (e.g., high arched or cleft palate), and note the movement of the uvula.

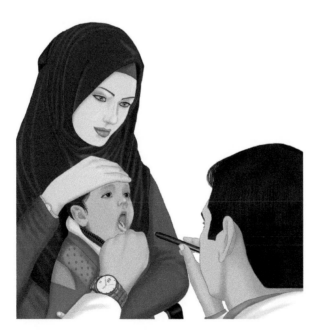

Fig. 4.12 Method of examination of the oral cavity by using a tongue depressor and a penlight.
© Anwar Qais Saadoon

4.8.3 Neck Examination

- **Inspection**
  - Inspect the symmetry and contour of the neck, and look for any abnormalities, such as a short, webbed neck (as in Turner syndrome), torticollis, swellings, or masses.
  - Ask the older child to swallow, and observe any abnormalities or masses that move with swallowing.
  - Note any scar, sinus, fistula, pulsation, or dilated veins.
  - Positioning the child at 45°, observe venous pulsation.
- **Range of movement**
  - Note the range of movement by having the child flex, extend, rotate, and laterally turn his/her head and neck. Note if the child has any pain or limitation in the movements, and observe whether the movements are smooth.
- **Palpation**
  - Ask the child to sit, and start the neck palpation from behind.
  - Palpate the neck from different sides, and flex the child's head to the side that is being palpated, looking for any abnormalities (such as masses or a goiter).
  - Palpate the neck while the muscles are being contracted by asking the child to resist your movement.
  - Palpate the trachea (it should be in midline position), cervical lymph nodes, and carotid arteries, feeling for any thrill.

Clinical Tips 4.7

If you detect a neck mass:
- Note its location:
  - A midline mass may suggest a thyroglossal cyst or goiter.
  - A lateral mass may suggest a lymph node, branchial cyst, cystic hygroma, or sternomastoid tumor.
- Examine its relation to different structures, such as the trachea and hyoid bone, noting movement with protruding of the tongue and with swallowing.
- Perform the transillumination test to see whether it is cystic or not.

4.9 Cardiovascular System Examination

- Following a systematic approach to the examination of cardiovascular system may be helpful (see Examination Station 4.3), but flexibility in the examination and taking advantage of opportunities are also required. It is a good practice to tailor the sequence and extent of the examination to the child's age and condition.
- Infants and toddlers are better to be examined on the parent's lap. They should be undressed to the diaper.
- Examine the older children and adolescents, with the patient sitting up on the examination table at 45° with head supported and body undressed to waist (with consideration for modesty in adolescents).

Examination Station 4.3: Cardiovascular System Examination

1. **General Physical Examination**
   - General inspection
   - Skin
     - Skin rash
     - Subcutaneous nodules
   - Face
     - Dysmorphic features
     - Cyanosis (central)
     - Pallor, polycythemia, and jaundice
     - Sweating
     - Oral hygiene and dental caries
   - Hands
     - Clubbing
     - Other signs that may suggest infective endocarditis:
       Splinter hemorrhages
       Osler's nodes
       Janeway's lesions
     - Cyanosis (peripheral)
     - Bony abnormalities
   - Pulses
   - Respiratory rate
   - Blood Pressure
   - Temperature
   - Oxygen saturation
   - Neck
     - Jugular venous pulse
     - Cervical lymphadenopathy
     - Trachea
   - Capillary refill
   - Abdomen: Examine for hepatosplenomegaly and ascites
   - Back and lower limbs
     - Look for edema and arthritis
   - Nervous system
   - Nutritional status assessment and anthropometric measures
2. **Examination of the Precordium**
   - **Inspection**
     - Depth of respiration, signs of respiratory distress
     - Scars of past surgery
     - Asymmetry
     - Visible ventricular impulse
     - Hyperdynamic precordium
     - Dilated veins

Continued on the next page

- **Palpation**
  - Apex beat
  - Heaves
  - Thrills
  - Palpable heart sounds
- **Percussion**
- **Auscultation**
  - Auscultate carefully over the four valve areas (see Fig. 4.13) and listen to:
    First and second heart sounds
    Added sounds, such as gallop rhythm in heart failure and ejection click in aortic stenosis
    Murmurs

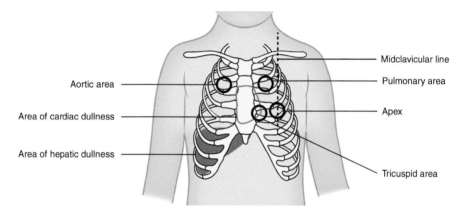

Aortic area

Area of cardiac dullness

Area of hepatic dullness

Midclavicular line

Pulmonary area

Apex

Tricuspid area

Fig. 4.13 Areas of heart auscultation

4.9.1   General Physical Examination

- **General inspection**
  - Look at the child and note whether he/she is well, irritable, lethargic, unconscious, dyspneic, etc.
  - Note whether the child takes a special position, e.g., squatting position in older children with tetralogy of Fallot (TOF). This position can decrease the amount of right-to-left shunting, and as a result, it increases systemic oxygen saturation.
- **Skin**
  - **Skin rash** (e.g., systemic lupus erythematosus (SLE) and Kawasaki disease)
  - **Subcutaneous nodules**, as in rheumatic fever.
  - Look for skin manifestations of syndromes that may be associated with cardiac conditions (e.g., Down syndrome or Turner syndrome).

- **Face**
  - **Dysmorphic features:** Cardiac disorders are more common in children with certain syndromes, for example:

    Atrial septal defect (ASD) and ventricular septal defect (VSD) are common in children with Down syndrome.

    Coarctation of the aorta is more common in children with Turner syndrome.

    Aortic incompetence is seen more in those with Marfan syndrome [34].
  - **Cyanosis**

    Examine the tongue, mucosa of the mouth, conjunctivae, skin, and lips for central cyanosis (see Box 4.6).

Box 4.6: Cyanosis

- Cyanosis is a bluish discoloration of the skin, mucous membranes, or nail beds.
- Involvement of the mucous membrane is very important in differentiation between central and peripheral cyanosis.
- **Central cyanosis:** Affects the oral mucosa, tongue, conjunctivae, skin, and lips. Its presence is always abnormal and may occur due to a variety of cardiac, pulmonary, and neurological diseases (e.g., hypoventilation); it may also occur in conditions of abnormal hemoglobin or acute methemoglobinemia.
- **Peripheral cyanosis:** Affects the skin and lips but spares the oral mucosa, tongue, and conjunctivae. The distal extremities, or sometimes the circumoral or periorbital areas, and ears are typically affected. This type of cyanosis happens in the presence of normal systemic arterial saturation and usually occurs after exposure to cold or due to inadequate peripheral circulation.
- **Acrocyanosis:** Refers to the peripheral cyanosis of the hands and feet, and around the mouth, caused by peripheral vasoconstriction and increased tissue oxygen extraction; it most commonly presents in the first 24 h of life as a normal observation.
- **Differential cyanosis** is a bluish discoloration of the lower limbs only, while the upper limbs remain pink. It points to right-to-left shunting across a ductus arteriosus in association with an interrupted aortic arch or coarctation of the aorta.
- **Reverse differential cyanosis** is blueness of the upper limbs, while the lower limbs are pink; it occurs in cases of transposition of the great arteries (TGA) with coarctation of aorta [35].

  - **Pallor, polycythemia, and jaundice**

    Pallor: Examine for pallor in the conjunctivae, oral mucosa, and lips. It usually indicates the presence of anemia, which can cause tachycardia or murmur; it also may point to poor peripheral perfusion.

Polycythemia often occurs with cyanotic congenital heart diseases.

Jaundice may occur due to hemolysis caused by a prosthetic heart valve.

– **Sweating**

Sweating during feedings should raise the concern for congestive heart failure, especially if it is associated with subcostal indrawing and rapid tiredness [36].

– **Oral hygiene and dental caries**

Poor oral hygiene and dental caries may lead to bacteremia, resulting in infective endocarditis.

• **Hand**

– **Clubbing:** clubbing of fingers and toes occurs in cyanotic congenital heart diseases after 6 months of age; it also can be seen in case of infective endocarditis. (See Table 4.7 and Box 4.3.)

– **Other signs that may suggest infective endocarditis:**

Splinter hemorrhages: tiny linear hemorrhages tend to run vertically underneath the nail

Osler's nodes: small, painful erythematous nodules found on the pads of the fingers and toes

Janeway's lesions: small, non-tender erythematous maculopapular lesions on the palm or sole

– **Cyanosis** (peripheral)

Examine the nail beds for peripheral cyanosis, which may indicate inadequate peripheral circulation (see Box 4.6).

– **Bony abnormalities,** such as an absent thumb or absent radii, are associated with certain syndromes that may point to cardiac diseases [37].

• **Pulses**

– Assess the peripheral pulses in all four extremities:

Palpate brachial and radial pulses (see below).

Palpate femoral pulses to exclude coarctation of the aorta.

Method of Palpation

Brachial pulse (preferred for children younger than 3 years)

– To feel the brachial pulse, flex the child's elbow partially, and use the first and second fingers (or the thumb) of your right hand, applied to the front of the elbow, just medial to the biceps tendon [36].

Radial pulse (preferred for older children)

– Palpate it, using the tips of your index and middle fingers, just lateral to the flexor carpi radialis tendon and proximal to the wrist on the thumb side.

– Assess for radio-radial delay by palpation of both radial pulses at the same time. By this method, you also can detect any difference in pulse volume [38].

Femoral pulse

– The child should lie flat on his/her back with a partially flexed knee; the hip should be abducted and externally rotated.

– Use the bulbs of your fingers to feel the femoral pulse just below the mid-inguinal point (the point which is located between the anterior superior iliac spine and the pubic symphysis).

- Routinely palpate the radial and femoral pulses at the same time to detect any delay or volume differences.
- A radio-femoral delay, or an absent or weak femoral pulse, may point to coarctation of the aorta [38].

By palpation of the right brachial pulse, assess the following:
Pulse rate: Count it over 30 s and multiply by 2 to find the beats per minute.
- Normal pulse rate: varies with the child's age (see Table 4.5).
- Tachycardia: Sinus tachycardia may be seen in an anxious or feverish child.
- Bradycardia: may be seen in complete heart block, junior athletes, and certain medications (such as beta-blockers).
Rhythm
- Regular (e.g., respiratory sinus arrhythmia), which is common in <u>young children</u>
- Regular irregularity (e.g., coupled extrasystoles)
- Irregular irregularity (e.g., atrial fibrillation, multiple extrasystoles)
Character: refers to the shape or waveform of the arterial pulse; it may be:
- Normal character
- Collapsing pulse, as in patent ductus arteriosus or aortic incompetence
- Slow rising pulse suggests left ventricular outflow tract obstruction
- Others: pulsus paradoxus, pulsus bisferiens, rapidly rising, ill-sustained, jerk, etc [37].
Volume (pulse pressure)
Pulse volume may be normal, small, large, or varying.
- Small volume occurs in heart failure, shock, or cardiac outflow abstraction.
- Large volume can be felt in anemia, fever, hyperthyroidism, aortic insufficiency, carbon dioxide retention, or patent ductus arteriosus [20].
- Varying volume may be seen in extrasystoles, atrial fibrillation, or incomplete heart block.
- **Respiratory rate**
  - Count the respiratory rate over 1 full minute. Tachypnea and respiratory distress occur in many cardiac conditions (e.g., heart failure).
- **Blood pressure**
  - Blood pressure should be measured in the arms and legs to exclude coarctation of the aorta (see Sect. 4.6.4).
- **Temperature**
  - Fever may indicate infection (e.g., viral myocarditis, rheumatic fever, nasopharyngitis, pneumonia, urinary tract infection, etc.).
- **Oxygen saturation**
  - Measure pre- and post-ductal oxygen saturations (see Chap. 3).
- **Neck**
  - **Jugular venous pulse**
    With the child reclining at 45°, inspect the neck for a prominent jugular venous pulsation, which suggests tricuspid incompetence, while cannon waves suggest a heart block.
  - **Cervical lymphadenopathy**

Significant cervical lymphadenopathy may occur in certain conditions with cardiac involvement (e.g., Kawasaki disease).

- **Trachea**

  Palpate the trachea and look for any deviation.

- **Capillary refill**
  - Apply blanching pressure with a finger or thumb on the skin of the child's sternum (or a digit at the heart level) <u>for 5 s, then release</u> and watch for the color to return. Blush normally takes <u>less than 2 s to return</u>; if it takes longer, then poor peripheral perfusion or shock should be suspected [21].

- **Abdomen**
  - Palpate and percuss the abdomen for hepatosplenomegaly; this may be a late sign of heart failure. The liver may be pushed downward in some respiratory conditions (e.g., bronchiolitis, pleural effusion, empyema, emphysema, etc.). Therefore, measurement of the liver span is very important to differentiate an enlarged liver from a pushed-down liver.
  - Enlargement of the spleen alone may occur in infective endocarditis.
  - Examine for ascites if heart failure is suspected.

- **Back and lower limbs**
  - Examine for edema (ankle, sacrum, and precordium).

    Pitting peripheral edema is a late manifestation of congestive heart failure in children [36].

    In infants, edema is usually seen periorbital and over the flanks, while in older children pedal edema occurs as well.
  - Examine for arthritis and look for joint swelling and skeletal deformities, which may point to syndromes or diseases that are associated with cardiac conditions (e.g., Marfan syndrome, systemic lupus erythematosus (SLE), or rheumatoid arthritis).

- **Nervous system**
  - Note any involuntary movements and focal deficits.

- **Nutritional status assessment and anthropometric measures**
  - Both heart failure and cyanotic congenital heart disease can lead to a failure to thrive. Hence, assessment of the nutritional status of the child, along with measurement of his/her growth parameters and plotting the readings on standard percentile growth charts, is very important [39].

4.9.2 Examination of the Precordium

- **Inspection**
  - Note the **depth of respiration and any signs of respiratory distress**, which may associate with cardiac diseases.
  - **Scars of past surgery**

    Look for scar of median sternotomy (which suggests that open-heart surgery has been performed) and left or right lateral thoracotomy (which suggests Blalock–Taussig or PDA ligation). Scars may be hidden under the arm or at the back.

- **Asymmetry**
  While the child is lying supine, inspect for asymmetry from the child's feet on the same plane as his/her chest. A left precordial bulge may indicate cardiomegaly [37].
- **Visible ventricular impulse**
  The left ventricular impulse (apex beat) can be seen in thin children or those with hyperdynamic circulation (e.g., excitement or fever), and it is also seen in left ventricular enlargement.
- **Hyperdynamic precordium**
  A hyperdynamic precordium may be normal in a thin child, or it may suggest a volume load (as in a large left-to-right shunt) [39].
- **Dilated veins over chest wall**
- **Palpation**
  - **Apex beat**
    Palpate for the apex beat with a flat hand or with the pulp of two fingers.
    In children aged <u>less than 4 years</u>, palpate for the apex beat <u>at the fourth intercostal space, slightly outside or at the left mid-clavicular line</u> (a vertical imaginary line passes through the midpoint of the clavicle.) In children <u>between 4 and 7 years</u>, the apex beat is located <u>in the fourth or fifth intercostal space at or slightly medial to the left mid-clavicular line</u>.
    In certain circumstances, the apex beat may be displaced from its normal place to the left (e.g., cardiomegaly) or to the right (e.g., congenital dextrocardia).
    Assess the character of the apex beat, as it may provide a vital diagnostic clue. For example:
    Sustained suggests pressure overload (e.g., aortic stenosis).
    Forceful indicates left ventricular hypertrophy.
    Thrusting points to volume overload (e.g., left-to-right shunt, mitral or aortic regurgitation).
    Tapping may occur in mitral stenosis.
    The apex beat may be absent in obese children or those with a hyperinflated chest, as well as in those who have pericardial effusion. Dextrocardia should also be considered.
  - **Heaves**
    A heave is a palpable impulse that prominently lifts your hand.
    Palpate for the left parasternal heave by placing the palm or the ulnar border of your right hand firmly over the left parasternal area. A presence of heave suggests right ventricular hypertrophy [37].
  - **Thrills**
    A thrill is a palpable murmur. Palpate for thrills with the flat of your hand over the apex, lower-left sternal edge (ventricular septal defect), upper-left sternal edge (pulmonary stenosis), upper-right sternal edge, and in the suprasternal notch (aortic stenosis or coarctation of the aorta).
  - **Palpable heart sounds**
    A palpable second heart sound may indicate pulmonary hypertension.

- **Percussion**
  - Percussion is inaccurate for assessing heart size in children, but it may be useful in detecting a mediastinal shift.
- **Auscultation**
  - The child should be quiet during the auscultation.
  - Use both the bell and the diaphragm of your stethoscope to listen carefully over the four valve areas (see Fig. 4.13):

  Apex

  Lower-left sternal edge (tricuspid area)

Table 4.8 Types of pathological murmurs in common heart diseases [28, 35–37, 39]

Lesion	Type of murmur	Best site to be heard	Radiation
Aortic stenosis	Ejection systolic	Aortic area (right second intercostal space)	Toward upper-right sternal edge, over carotids
Pulmonary stenosis	Ejection systolic	Pulmonary area (left second intercostal space)	To left side of the neck or beneath left scapula
Atrial septal defect (ASD)	Ejection systolic with a wide, fixed splitting of the second heart sound	Pulmonary area	To right axilla
Aortic incompetence	Early diastolic	Upper and mid-left sternal border (best heard while the child is sitting and holding on expiration)	Down left sternal edge toward apex, left axilla
Pulmonary incompetence	Early diastolic	Left sternal border	
Mitral stenosis (rare)	Mid-diastolic	Apex	
Tricuspid stenosis	Mid-diastolic	Apex	
Mitral incompetence	Pansystolic	Apex	To left axilla or beneath left scapula
Tricuspid incompetence	Pansystolic	Lower-left sternal border	To epigastrium or to lower-right sternal border
Ventricular septal defect (VSD)	Pansystolic with mid-diastolic (if large)	Lower-left sternal border (fourth intercostal space)	All over pericardium
Mitral valve prolapse	Late systolic	Apex	
Patent ductus arteriosus (PDA)	Continuous	Left second intercostal space	To back and left clavicle
Coarctation of the aorta	Systolic or continuous	Left sternal border	To left infrascapular area and occasionally to the neck

Upper-left sternal edge (pulmonary area)

Upper-right sternal edge (aortic area)

- If you heard a murmur over any of these areas, listen over the site of radiation (see Table 4.8).
- Do not forget to auscultate over the back for patent ductus arteriosus (PDA), pulmonary stenosis (PS), and coarctation of the aorta.
- Auscultate with the child in both lying and sitting positions, and concentrate on the following:

Heart Sounds

- **First heart sound**
  - The first heart sound results from the closure of mitral and tricuspid valves.
  - A loud first heart sound is heard in:

    Atrial septal defect (ASD)

    Mechanical prosthetic valve

    Mitral stenosis (rarely)

- **Second heart sound**
  - The second heart sound results from closure of aortic and pulmonary valves.
  - A loud second heart sound is heard in:

    Conditions that lead to increased pulmonary flow, such as patent ductus arteriosus (PDA), atrial septal defect (ASD), and large ventricular septal defect (VSD)

    Pulmonary hypertension

  - It is important to note any changes in heart sounds with breathing. Splitting of the second heart sound may normally occur with respiration, but a wide fixed (i.e., invariable with breathing) splitting may point to an atrial septal defect (ASD).

Added Sounds

- **Third heart sound**
  - A low-pitched sound may be heard early in diastole after the second heart sound. It is best heard with the bell of the stethoscope at the apex.
  - It is normally heard in healthy infants and younger children, but it can also be heard in heart failure.
- **Fourth heart sound**
  - A fourth heart sound may be heard just before the first heart sound.
  - It is always pathological and may indicate pulmonary hypertension or heart failure.
- **Opening snap**
  - An opening snap is a high-pitched sound that may be heard after the second heart sound and may point to mitral stenosis.
- **Ejection click**
  - An ejection click is a high-pitched sound that may be heard early in systole after the first heart sound and may indicate aortic or pulmonary stenosis.

Murmurs
- Murmurs are sounds caused by the turbulence of blood flow. They may be innocent or pathological.
- If you hear a murmur, check for the following:
  - **Timing**: systolic, diastolic, or continuous
    Diastolic murmurs are always pathological.
  - **Duration**: early diastolic, late systolic, pansystolic, etc.
  - **Grading of murmurs**:
    Grade I—barely audible
    Grade II—medium intensity
    Grade III—easily heard, but no thrill
    Grade IV—loud with a thrill

Notes 4.9

- Grades I and II are usually innocent murmurs. Grades V and VI are always significant.

    Grade V—very loud with a thrill, often heard over a wide area
    Grade VI—extremely loud with a thrill. It can be heard even without a
       stethoscope
  - **Pitch**: low-pitched murmurs may be caused by a large opening, a low-pressure gradient, or both, while high-pitched murmurs may result from a small opening, a high-pressure gradient, or both.
  - **Quality**: blowing, harsh, musical, or rumbling.
  - **Site of maximum intensity and radiation** (see Table 4.8).

Normal Murmurs (Innocent)
- Normal murmurs are common in children, due to increased blood flow velocity. They can be distinguished from pathological murmurs by the fact that they are usually systolic, soft, and short, with a musical quality, without radiation, and symptom-free, with no abnormal signs or tests.

Pathological Murmurs (See Table 4.8)
- These are generally of high grades (≥3), with a harsh quality; they may radiate to other sites and may be symptomatic and associated with abnormal signs and tests. They can be classified as:
  - Systolic murmurs
  - Diastolic murmurs
  - Continuous murmurs

4.10   Respiratory System Examination

- Respiratory tract infection is the main cause of seeking medical attention in children. Therefore, it is wise to give more attention to the examination of the respiratory system.
- Infants and toddlers are best examined on their parent's lap. This may keep them calm.
- Older children or adolescents should be positioned at 45–60° on the examination table with head supported and body exposed to waist (with sensitivity toward modesty in young adults).

Examination Station 4.4: Respiratory System Examination

1. **General Physical Examination**
   - **General inspection**
     - General health and activity
     - Nutritional status and level of consciousness
     - Color
     - Position of comfort
     - Noisy breathing: wheeze, stridor, and grunting
     - Voice changes and cough (inspect any sputum)
   - **Face**
     - Dysmorphic features
     - Cyanosis
     - Pallor
     - Traumatic petechiae
     - Nasal discharge
   - **Neck**
     - Tracheal tug
     - Swelling, cystic hygroma, goiter
   - **Hands**
     - Clubbing
2. **Examination of the Chest**
   - **Inspection**
     - Shape
     - Chest wall abnormalities and deformities
       Harrison's sulcus
       Rachitic rosary
     - Asymmetry
     - Scars
     - Movement
     - Breathing pattern
     - Respiratory rate
     - Signs of respiratory distress

Continued on the next page

- **Palpation**
  - Mediastinal deviation
    Tracheal deviation
    Apex beat
  - Chest expansion
  - Tactile vocal fremitus
- **Percussion**
- **Auscultation**
  - Air entry
  - Breath sounds: vesicular, bronchovesicular, or bronchial breath sounds
  - Added sounds
    Transmitted upper-airway sounds
    Rhonchi
    Crackles
    Pleural friction rub
  - Vocal resonance
    Bronchophony (bronchiloquy)
    Whispering pectoriloquy
    Egophony

4.10.1 General Physical Examination

- **General inspection**
  - **General health and activity**
    Observe the child's health and activity, because some respiratory diseases may interfere with the child's activity and may affect his/her general health (e.g., asthma).
  - **Nutritional status and level of consciousness**
    Some respiratory diseases may associate with failure to thrive, such as cystic fibrosis. Therefore, assessment of the nutritional status of the child is of value [21].
    Assess the consciousness level of the child, noting any restlessness or drowsiness, which may be associated with acute respiratory distress [34].
  - **Color:** Baby's color may provide a clue to his/her general condition.
  - **Position of comfort**
    Children tend to take a particular position to alleviate airway obstruction in some respiratory diseases—e.g., tripod position which may be seen in the case of acute epiglottitis.
  - **Noisy breathing**
    A wheeze is a continuous musical sound usually heard during expiration, as in bronchiolitis or asthma.

Stridor is a harsh, high-pitched inspiratory noise caused by obstruction of the airway between the nose and the larger bronchi.

Grunting is a repetitive, short expiratory sound, which results from expiration against closed epiglottis, and it may indicate a significant respiratory disease.

- **Voice changes and cough**
  Changes in a child's voice may provide a clue about certain diseases. (For example, "rocks in the mouth" suggest tonsillitis, while hoarse voice with cough may indicate croup.)
  If you hear a cough, try to know its character.
  If there is sputum, inspect it carefully.

- **Face**
  - **Dysmorphic features** may suggest certain syndromes that can affect respiratory system e.g., Down syndrome, which may be associated with sleep apnea syndrome.
  - **Cyanosis** may indicate respiratory failure (see Box 4.6).
  - **Pallor:** Look at lower palpebral conjunctiva for pallor.
  - **Traumatic petechiae** may occur over the face, eyelids, or neck after a bout of severe coughing.
  - **Nasal discharge** is a common presentation in upper-respiratory tract infection. It also may occur in case of the presence of a foreign body in the nose [21].

- **Neck**
  - **Tracheal tug:** Rest your fingers on the child's trachea. They may move inferiorly with each inspiration. This may indicate severe hyperinflation.
  - **Swelling, cystic hygroma, and goiter:** These may interfere with the child's breathing.

- **Hands**
  - **Clubbing of fingers** can be seen in chronic suppurative lung disease (e.g., bronchiectasis, lung abscess, empyema, and cystic fibrosis) or cyanotic congenital heart disease (e.g., tetralogy of Fallot). (See Table 4.7 and Box 4.3.)

4.10.2 Examination of the Chest

1. **Inspection**
   (a) **Shape:** Look for any abnormal chest shape—e.g., pectus excavatum (funnel chest) or pectus carinatum (pigeon chest).
   (b) **Chest wall abnormalities and deformities**
     - Harrison's sulcus
       - Costal cartilages are retracted, with flaring lower ribs at the costal margin. It may suggest chronic airway obstruction or left-to-right cardiac shunt [37].
     - Rachitic rosary
       - Costochondral junction swelling, which may occur in rickets, in scurvy, and sometimes in achondroplasia

(c) **Asymmetry**
(d) **Scars:** Look for scars of median sternotomy or left or right thoracotomy, and carefully inspect for scars of previous chest drains.
(e) **Movement:** Compare movement of both sides of the chest in the full respiratory cycle.
(f) **Breathing pattern**
   • Rapid, shallow respiration with prolonged expiration occurs in asthma or bronchiolitis.
   • Kussmaul respirations (rapid, regular, deap, sighing respirations) suggest metabolic acidosis (e.g., diabetic ketoacidosis).
   • Cheyne–Stokes respirations: respirations with increasing and then decreasing depth and rate, alternating with periods of apnea or hypopnea.
(g) **Respiratory rate:** Count the respiratory rate within 1 full minute, and see whether it is normal for the given age (see Box 4.7).

Box 4.7: Tachypnea

• Tachypnea can be defined as an abnormally increased respiratory rate.
• According to the World Health Organization (WHO), the cutoff line for tachypnea in different age groups is as follows:
   – >60 breaths/min in infants aged less than 2 months
   – >50 breaths/min in infants aged 2 months to 1 year
   – >40 breaths/min in children older than 1 year of age [1]

(h) **Watch for signs of respiratory distress** (see Table 4.9):
   • Tachypnea and tachycardia
   • Nasal flaring
   • Grunting, wheezing, or stridor
   • Chest recessions/retractions (subcostal, intercostal, suprasternal)
   • Tracheal tug
   • Hyperinflation
   • Use of accessory muscles of respiration (mainly the sternocleidomastoid, scalene, and abdominal muscles); note any head bobbing in babies.
   • Abdominal paradoxical movement
   • Cyanosis and pallor
   • Difficulty in speaking, drinking, or walking
   • Hypotension

Table 4.9 Grades of respiratory distress [40, 41]

Mild	Moderate	Severe
• Tachypnea • Mild chest recessions/ retractions • Feeding and speech are not affected	• Tachypnea • Recessions are moderate or severe • Struggles to feed • Cannot speak in full sentences	• Tachycardia • Gasping • Head bobbing • Inability to speak • Frightened • Cyanotic, pale • Quiet or agitated • Hypoxic, even with oxygen • Chest may be silent • Consciousness may be impaired

2. **Palpation**
   (a) Palpation and percussion are not done routinely in infants or younger children.
   (b) You can do them in particular situations, such as:
       • Assessment of hyperinflation
       • Detection of the upper border of the liver
       • Confirmation of signs of collapse, consolidation, or effusion
   (c) **Mediastinal deviation**
       • **Tracheal deviation**
         – Palpate the trachea in the suprasternal notch by using your index finger. Tracheal deviation to any side indicates certain pathology (e.g., tension pneumothorax, unilateral effusion, or thoracic mass) [35].
       • **Apex beat**
         – Use your palm to localize the apex beat at the fourth intercostal space in the mid-clavicular line.
         – A mediastinal shift (e.g., pneumothorax or pleural effusion) can lead to apex beat displacement [35, 38].
   (d) **Chest expansion**
       • Assess maximum chest expansion from the front by placing your hands firmly on the child's chest.
       • Your fingers should just grasp the sides of the child's chest, and your outstretched thumbs should be at the level of the nipples and just touch each other at the midline, but they should not touch the chest.
       • Ask the child to take a deep, big breath after full inhalation and exhalation.
       • Your thumbs will act as "calipers." The distance your thumbs move symmetrically away from each other during inspiration determines the degree of chest expansion. It is usually about 3–5 cm in school-aged children [1, 20].
       • To measure chest expansion posteriorly, repeat the same method on the child's back, but your thumbs should be at T10 level.
       • Hyperinflation and restrictive lung disease can reduce chest expansion symmetrically.

(e) **Tactile vocal fremitus**
  - Fremitus means the palpable vibrations transmitted through the bronchi and bronchioles to the chest wall as the child is speaking [28].
  - If the child is aged more than 5 years, ask him/her to repeat "ninety-nine" while you place the palmar bases of your fingers (or the ulnar aspect of both hands) on either side of the chest. Feel for vibrations, comparing side to side and repeat the same posteriorly.
  - In a crying infant, you can assess vocal fremitus by palpation of the transmitted sounds over the chest [1].
  - Vocal fremitus may be increased as in consolidation, decreased as in collapse, or absent as in pleural effusion [35, 37].

3. **Percussion**
  (a) Explain to the child what you are going to do.
  (b) Percussion should be gentle.
  (c) Press firmly on the surface to be percussed, using your left middle finger (it should be hyperextended), and then strike its middle phalanx by the tip of your right middle finger at a right angle to it.
  (d) Movement of your hand should be quick, sharp, and coming from the wrist.
  (e) Avoid any other contacts between your hands and the child's chest.
  (f) Percuss anteriorly and posteriorly, and start from the upper to lower chest.
  (g) Compare side by side.
  (h) Percuss the clavicle directly.
  (i) A normal lung gives a resonant percussion note; a hyperresonant note suggests pneumothorax or emphysema; a dull note may indicate consolidation, collapse, fibrosis, or pleural thickening; a stony, dull note suggests effusion [5].

4. **Auscultation**
  (a) If the child is old enough, tell him/her what you are going to do.
  (b) Do not start auscultation through the clothing.
  (c) Use the bell or diaphragm of a pediatric stethoscope for auscultation. The low-pitched sounds of the chest are better heard with the bell. Furthermore, the bell is smaller and warmer than the diaphragm, and it allows less surface noise [1].
  (d) Ask the child to breathe through his/her mouth.
  (e) Auscultate anteriorly and in the axillae, comparing side to side while listening from the upper to the lower chest.
  (f) Repeat the auscultation from the back in a similar way.
  (g) Try to assess the following:
    - *Air entry:* Is the air entry bilaterally equal?
    - *Breath sounds:* Assess the quality and amplitude of the breath sounds, identifing the length of inspiratory and expiratory phases and the presence of any gap between them.
      - *Normal breath sounds are vesicular*
        Low-pitched sounds, with no distinct interval between inspiration and expiration

- **Bronchovesicular breath sounds (prolonged expiration)**
  Similar to vesicular, no gap between inspiration and expiration but characterized by a prolonged expiration
  Suggests bronchopneumonias, asthma, or emphysema
- **Bronchial breath sounds**
  High-pitched sounds with a tubular quality, characterized by equal inspiratory and expiratory phases with a gap in between
  Suggests consolidation, fibrosis, or atelectasis
- **Diminished or absent breath sounds**
  May suggest a bronchial obstruction, severe bronchitis, collapse pleural effusion, pneumothorax, or a foreign-body inhalation.
- *Added Sounds*
  - **Transmitted upper-airway sounds**
    These are harsh sounds transmitted from the upper airway to the chest, such as gurgling. They are common in infants and toddlers [1, 37].
    If you hear coarse, variable crackles in the chest, placing your stethoscope on the side of the child's neck may help you to know whether these sounds are transmitted or not. The conducted sounds will be louder over the neck [37].
  - **Rhonchi**
    Continuous, musical, high-pitched expiratory sounds indicate narrowing of the distal airway, due to mucosal edema, excessive mucus, or bronchospasm [1].
  - **Crackles** (rales formally)
    Discontinuous, non-musical, moist sounds result from the opening and closing of the bronchioles. Crackles may be fine or coarse.
    Fine inspiratory crackles suggest an alveolar or bronchiolar disease, such as pulmonary edema or fibrosing alveolitis.
    Coarse inspiratory or expiratory crackles can be heard in pneumonia or bronchiectasis.
    If you heard crackles, ask the child to cough, and recheck to hear whether it is cleared or not.
  - **Pleural friction rub**
    A loud creaking sound indicates pleural irritation, as in pleurisy.
    It is uncommon in children [37].
- *Vocal Resonance*
  - Vocal resonance refers to the character of the patient's voice that is heard over his/her chest with the stethoscope.
  - If the child is old enough, ask him/her to say, "ninety-nine" while you auscultate his/her chest. Listen to the areas of the chest symmetrically to assess the amplitude and quality of vocal resonance.
  - Normally, the patient's voice is heard faintly and indistinctly. It becomes louder and clearer over areas of consolidation.

– The changes in vocal resonance that may be seen in certain diseases are:
Bronchophony (bronchiloquy): The patient's voice is heard louder than normal over areas of consolidation.
Whispering pectoriloquy
Ask the child to whisper "ninety-nine" while you are listening over the auscultation areas. If the voice becomes louder and clearer, this is called "whispering pectoriloquy," which occurs in the case of airless lungs, such as lobar pneumonia [28, 37].
Egophony
Ask the child to say "ee" while you are listening over the area of abnormally located bronchial or bronchovesicular breath sounds. In some cases, such as lobar pneumonia, the voice will be heard as "ay" (as in say) [28, 37].
– Vocal resonance provides the same information as vocal fremitus, so it is sufficient to perform one of them [37].

4.11 Gastrointestinal System Examination

• The gastrointestinal system examination is an important component of pediatric physical examination. A comprehensive examination is discussed in this section. However, in practice, your examination should be guided by the patient's history and your observations.
• Confirmation of the child's age is very important as it helps you to focus your examination and to narrow the differential diagnosis.
• Place the child in a suitable position: supine on the parent's lap (for infants) or on the examination table (for older children).

Examination Station 4.5: Gastrointestinal System Examination

1. **General Physical Examination**
   • **General inspection**
     – General observations (e.g., intravenous fluid, nasogastric, or gastrostomy tube)
     – General health and level of consciousness
     – Hydration status
     – Nutritional status and growth
   • **Skin**
     – Skin rashes, bruising, scratch marks, or pigmentation
   • **Hands**
     – Clubbing of fingers
     – Koilonychia, leukonychia
     – Palmar erythema, pallor
     – Wide wrists

Continued on the next page

- Asterixis (flapping tremor)
- Xanthoma
- **Head and neck**
  - Face
    Dysmorphic features
    Spider nevi
  - Eyes
    Xanthelasma
    Jaundice and pallor
    Kayser–Fleischer rings
  - Mouth
    Gross abnormalities, abnormal odors, abnormal pigmentations, angular stomatitis, ulcers, gum hypertrophy, dental caries, poor oral hygiene
  - Neck
    Cervical lymphadenopathy
- **Chest**
  - Gynecomastia, spider nevi
2. **Examination of the Abdomen**
   - **Inspection**
     - Contour, distention, umbilicus
     - Scars, stomas, or striae
     - Movement with respiration
     - Masses, hernias, or hydroceles
     - Dilated veins, visible peristalsis
   - **Auscultation**
     - Bowel sounds
   - **Palpation**
     - Superficial palpation
     - Deep palpation
     - Organ palpation: liver, spleen, kidneys
     - Palpation for ascites
   - **Percussion**
     - **Organomegaly**
     - **Ascites**
3. **Further Examination**
   - **Groin:** hernias, diaper rash
   - **Genitalia**
   - **Examination of the abdomen posteriorly**
   - **Anus and rectum**
   - **Lower extremities:** erythema nodosum, clubbing, koilonychia, leukonychia

4.11.1 General Physical Examination

- **General inspection**
  - **General observations:** Inspect **around the bed**, looking for any clue that may help you in the assessment of the child's condition. Look for:
  Intravenous fluids
  Nutritional supplements: Note the presences of routes for enteral nutrition (e.g., nasogastric or gastrostomy) or parenteral nutrition (e.g., a central line)
  - **General health and level of consciousness**
  Note the general health of the child and see whether he/she is well or ill. This is helpful in the assessment of the severity of the disease.
  Assess the level of consciousness of the child because some gastrointestinal disorders can lead to a disturbed consciousness level, such as hepatic coma.
  - **Hydration state:** A child with diarrhea may have dehydration.
  - **Nutritional status and growth**
  Gastrointestinal diseases can cause malnutrition (e.g., malabsorption)
  Assessment of the growth parameters (weight, length or height, and head circumference) is very important, as many gastrointestinal diseases can lead to a failure to thrive.
- **Skin**
  - **Skin rashes:** Dermatitis herpetiformis suggests celiac disease.
  - **Bruising** may occur in liver dysfunction.
  - **Scratch marks** may suggest pruritus secondary to obstructive (cholestatic) jaundice.
  - **Pigmentation:** Look for depigmentation, hypopigmentation, or hyperpigmentation, as these may be associated with gastrointestinal diseases.
- **Hands**
  - **Clubbing of fingers** may be associated with gastrointestinal diseases (e.g., liver cirrhosis, inflammatory bowel disease, and malabsorption). (See Table 4.7 and Box 4.3.)
  - **Koilonychia:** Spoon-shaped nails suggest chronic iron deficiency.
  - **Leukonychia:** White-colored nails may indicate hypoalbuminemia (e.g., chronic liver disease, inflammatory bowel disease, celiac disease, or kwashiorkor).
  - **Palmar erythema** suggests chronic liver disease.
  - **Pallor**
  Inspect the palmar creases and nail beds for pallor.
  Pallor may suggest anemia, which may be caused by malabsorption or chronic gastrointestinal blood loss.
  - **Wide wrists** suggest rickets.
  - **Asterixis (flapping tremor):** Ask the child to extend his/her arms and dorsiflex the hands. Note any jerky movements in his/her hands, resembling a bird flapping its wings. Flapping tremor may occur in metabolic encephalopathy (e.g., liver failure, chronic renal failure, or acute respiratory failure).
  - **Xanthoma:** Lipid deposits cause tendon nodules or yellow skin. This may be seen in cases of hyperlipidemia (e.g., familial hypercholesterolemia).

- **Head and neck**
  - **Face**

    Dysmorphic features may indicate certain syndromes that may be associated with gut abnormalities (e.g., Down syndrome associated with duodenal atresia).

    Spider nevi (spider angiomas) are small (1–10 mm) cutaneous vascular malformations (visible end-arterioles beneath the skin surface), suggesting chronic liver disease.
  - **Eyes**

    Xanthelasma: Yellow plaques resulting from abnormal deposits of lipids around the eyes. They indicate an abnormal lipid profile.

    Jaundice and pallor

    Inspect the sclerae in natural light to detect any jaundice. It may be caused by liver diseases.

    Look at lower palpebral conjunctiva for pallor, which indicates anemia.

    Kayser–Fleischer rings are blue-green rings encircling the iris, caused by abnormal copper deposits. They occur in Wilson disease.
  - **Mouth**

    Note the general appearance of the mouth and jaw, then inspect inside the mouth, noting any:

    Gross abnormalities in the mouth and jaw, such as a cleft lip, which may interfere with the child's feeding

    Brown perioral pigmentation, suggesting Peutz–Jeghers syndrome

    Angular stomatitis and glossitis

    Abnormal odors (e.g., sweet-smelling breath suggests diabetic ketoacidosis)

    Gum hypertrophy, which may suggest myeloid leukemia or a side effect of using certain medications

    Poor oral hygiene and dental caries

    Ulcers (e.g., aphthous ulcers). Recurrent ulcers suggest inflammatory bowel diseases, Behcet disease, or celiac disease.

    Tonsillitis, which may be associated with abdominal pain
  - **Neck**

    Cervical lymphadenopathy: Significant cervical lymphadenopathy may indicate abdominal tuberculosis or lymphoma. Examine for hepatosplenomegaly if lymphoma is suspected.
- **Chest**
  - **Gynecomastia** may be normal but also may suggest chronic liver disease.
  - **Spider nevi:** The presence of multiple spider nevi (five or more) in the distribution of the superior vena cava may point to chronic liver disease.

4.11.2 Examination of the Abdomen

The abdomen can be divided into nine regions by two imaginary lines passing vertically through the mid-clavicular and the mid-inguinal points and two imaginary horizontal lines passing through the subcostal margins and anterior iliac crests (see Fig. 4.14).

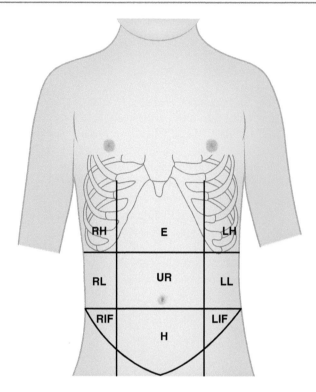

Fig. 4.14 The nine topographic regions of the abdomen: *LIF* left iliac fossa, *LL* left lumbar or flank region, *LH* left hypochondrium, *E* epigastrium, *RH* right hypochondrium, *RL* right lumbar or flank region, *RIF* right iliac fossa, *H* hypogastrium or suprapubic region, *UR* umbilical region

In infants or younger children, it may be sufficient to divide the abdomen into four quadrants by an imaginary horizontal line through the umbilicus and a vertical imaginary line from the xiphoid process to the symphysis pubis through the umbilicus (see Fig. 4.15). These regions or quadrants are of clinical importance as they help in the localization of any abnormality.

1. **Inspection**

   Bend both of the child's knees and inspect the abdomen, looking for:

   (a) **Contour**
       - Scaphoid, flat, or protuberant. The abdomen of toddlers is normally protuberant in erect posture, due to exaggerated lordosis.
       - Note any asymmetry.

   (b) **Distention**
       - See whether it is generalized or localized, symmetrical or not, or central or flank.
       - Abdominal distention may be caused by "the five Fs": fat, feces, flatus, fluid, or fetus (in adolescent female).

   (c) **Scars and striae**
       - Renal angle scars, liver biopsy, or laparoscopic surgery
       - Note any striae.

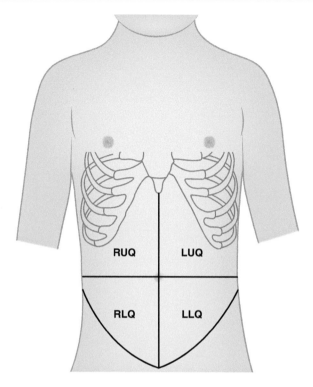

Fig. 4.15   The four quadrants of the abdomen: *LLQ* left lower quadrant, *LUQ* left upper quadrant, *RUQ* right upper quadrant, *RLQ* right lower quadrant

(d) **Stomas or drains:** Note any ileostomy, colostomy, or surgical drain.
(e) **Movement with respiration**
  - Up to school age, respiration of children is abdominal.
  - In certain conditions (e.g., peritonitis), the abdomen may not move freely with breathing.
(f) **Umbilicus:** Notice its position, shape, and whether there is any discharge.
(g) **Masses:** Masses or organomegaly may be obvious on inspection.
(h) **Hernias or hydroceles:** Ask the child to cough while inspecting the inguinal region and the scrotum for any visible swelling.
(i) **Dilated veins:** Dilated veins on the abdominal wall can be seen in cases of portal hypertension (especially periumbilical dilated veins) or vena cava obstruction (inferior or superior).
(j) **Visible peristalsis:** Visible peristalsis suggests intestinal obstruction.

2. **Auscultation**
  (a) Auscultation for bowel sounds should be done before the palpation or percussion because they can produce erratic bowel sounds.
  (b) Listen carefully for the bowel sounds by placing the warm diaphragm of your stethoscope over the center of the child's abdomen, to the right of the umbilicus, for up to 2 min.

    (c) The average frequency of bowel sounds is <u>6 per min</u>.

    (d) The absence of bowel sounds may suggest paralytic ileus or peritonitis.

    (e) Exaggerated bowel sounds may indicate acute infective diarrhea or intestinal obstruction.

    (f) Listen over any abdominal mass or palpable liver for bruits.

    (g) If the child has hypertension or neurofibromatosis, auscultate for renal bruits, as these conditions may be associated with renal artery stenosis.

3. **Palpation**

    (a) Ask the child to place his/her arms on the sides and flex both hips and knees to relax the abdominal muscles.

    (b) Ask the child whether there is a pain at any site of his/her abdomen. If there is a pain, ask the child to point to the site with one finger. Begin palpation with a warm hand away from that site, approaching the areas of the pain or lesion last.

    (c) If possible, ask the parents to help in diverting the child's

- **Superficial Palpation**
    - Get down to the child's level on the right side, and palpate all nine regions of the abdomen in turn. Start palpation in the left iliac fossa region, and move counterclockwise while watching the child's facial expression for any grimacing or wincing in response to tenderness. In addition, note any muscle guarding or superficial masses.
    - Examine for superficial swelling by asking the older child to contract his/her abdominal muscles or elevate his/her head while you are palpating the abdomen.
    - Ask the child to cough while you are palpating the hernial orifices to test for cough impulse.
    - If there are dilated veins, determine the direction of blood flow in the vein by pressing on the dilated vein with two fingers and pulling them apart; then lift one finger and watch the filling of the vein. The blood flows superiorly in case of inferior vena cava (IVC) obstruction and inferiorly when there is a superior vena cava (SVC) obstruction.
- **Deep palpation**
    - Ask the child to breathe in and out. Palpate the abdomen when the child breathes.
    - Repeat the same steps of superficial palpation, but palpate deeper with each relaxation period of respiration.
    - Note deep masses and deep tenderness; palpate deeply and quickly, and then release the pressure to detect any rebound tenderness that may suggest peritoneal irritation.
    - If you find any tenderness, determine its location.
    - If you find a mass, try to determine the following:
      Its location, size, and shape
      Consistency (an indentable mass on left iliac fossa may just be feces)
      Mobility on respiration
      Whether tender or not
      Its behavior during abdominal contraction

- **Organ palpation**

  Liver

  – Ask the child to breathe in and out.
  – Start the palpation from the right iliac fossa with the tips of your fingers; the fingers should point toward the child's head (see Fig. 4.16a).
  – Slide your fingers gradually, moving them up toward the costal margin until you feel the liver edge as it descends on inspiration.
  – Another method of liver palpation is by using the side of your right index finger with the left hand posteriorly in the right loin.
  – The liver edge is normally palpable below the costal margin (up to 2 cm) in neonates and (up to 1 cm) in children younger than 3 years.
  – If you find an enlarged liver, describe its position and texture, whether tender or not and whether pulsatile or expansile. Comment on its surface (smooth, nodular, or granular) and borders (rounded, sharp, or leafy).
  – Percuss over the upper edge of the liver to exclude hyperinflation as the cause of the palpable liver edge.
  – Use a tape measure to measure the liver span, measuring (in centimeters) the distance between the upper (by percussion) and lower (by palpation) edges of the liver in the mid-clavicular line. Normal liver span in infants is 6–10 cm, and it ranges from 6 to 12 cm in children aged 6–12 years.

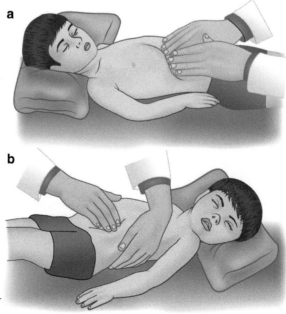

Fig. 4.16 Methods of palpation: (**a**) Liver and (**b**) Spleen

Spleen (see Fig. 4.16b)

- Ask the child to breathe deeply in and out.
- Start palpation with the tips of the fingers of your right hand from the right iliac fossa, moving your hand slowly up toward the left hypochondrium.
- Your left hand should splint the lower edge of the rib cage posteriorly.
- Percuss the spleen borders.
- Use a tape measure to measure the extent of the spleen below the costal margin in the mid-clavicular line.
- You may feel the spleen (1–2 cm) below the left costal margin of an infant. This is considered normal. Key causes of an enlarged spleen and/or liver are listed in Table 4.10.
- An enlarged spleen can be distinguished from the enlarged left kidney by the following:
  The spleen has a notch, while the kidney does not.
  You cannot feel above the spleen.
  Percussion over the spleen will give a dull note.
  The spleen is not ballottable, but the kidney is.

Kidneys

- Palpate for enlarged kidneys by placing one hand in the renal angle (the costovertebral angle) and the other one on the anterior of the child's abdomen, just lateral to the rectus abdominis muscle (see Fig. 4.17).
- Push both hands simultaneously (firmly, but gently), while the child breathes out, and ask him/her to take a deep breath; you will feel the movement of the lower pole of the enlarged kidney between your hands.

Table 4.10 Key causes of liver and spleen enlargement in children, with examples [21, 42]

Causes of hepatomegaly	Causes of splenomegaly	Causes of hepatosplenomegaly
• **Infectious diseases** Hepatitis A infection, malaria, or infectious mononucleosis	• **Hematological disorders** Hemolytic anemia (e.g., thalassemia major)	• **Lymphoma**
• **Hematological disorders** Thalassemia major	• **Infectious diseases** Kala-azar, brucellosis, infectious mononucleosis, or malaria	• **Myeloproliferative diseases**
• **Malignancies** Leukemia, lymphoma, hepatoblastoma, neuroblastoma, Wilms' tumor or other metastatic cancers	• **Malignancy** Acute leukemia or lymphoma	• **Cirrhosis with portal hypertension**
• **Cardiovascular diseases** Heart failure	• **Rheumatological conditions** Systemic lupus erythematosus or systemic juvenile idiopathic arthritis	• **Rare causes** Glycogen storage disease, amyloidosis, or sarcoidosis
• **Liver disease** Chronic active hepatitis	• **Other causes** Portal hypertension, glycogen storage disorders, amyloidosis	
• **Rare causes** Glycogen storage disorders or amyloidosis		

Fig. 4.17 Method of
kidney palpation in
children

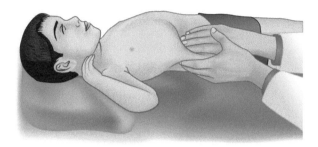

- If you felt the kidney, push it forward and backward; it should be ballottable.
- Assess the size, surface, and consistency of the palpable kidney.
- Kidneys may be palpable in <u>neonates</u> and <u>healthy, thin infants</u>.

Bladder
- Palpate for the bladder in the lower abdomen.
- The bladder may be palpable when full.

4. **Percussion**
   (a) Percuss the entire abdomen and listen to the percussion note. It is normally resonant; dull over an enlarged spleen, liver, a mass, or a full bladder; and hyperresonant over a distended bowel loop with gas.
   (b) In a cooperative child, percuss for the following:
   - **Organomegaly**
     Liver
     - Ask the older child to hold his/her breath on full expiration.
     - Percuss along the mid-clavicular line to identify the upper and lower liver borders.
     - Start percussion at the fourth intercostal space and move downward.
     - Normally, the liver dullness begins at the fifth intercostal space and continues just below the costal margin.

     Spleen
     - Percuss along the left anterior axillary line at the lowest intercostal space.
     - Ask the child to take a deep breath while you are percussing the area; it should stay resonant for the period of inspiration. If the percussion note changes from resonant to dull, splenomegaly should be suspected.

     Masses
     - Percuss over the mass.
     - The percussion note may be dull in solid or cystic masses or resonant if there is a bowel overlying the mass.

     Ascites
     - Check for ascites if there is any of the following:
       Distended abdomen with dullness over the flanks
       Signs of liver disease
       Hepatosplenomegaly
       Presence of edema
     - There are two main methods for assessing the presence of ascites: shifting dullness and fluid thrill.

Shifting Dullness
- With the child supine, percuss from the umbilicus toward the flanks, putting your fingers parallel to the flank and pointing toward the child's head.
- Keep the examining hand over the exact site where the percussion note changed from resonance to dullness.
- Ask the child to roll onto his/her opposite side. Wait for a while; the fluid will move to the lower flank.
- Repeat the percussion so the position of the dullness will be shifted.

Fluid Thrill
- When the abdomen is tensely distended, feel for the fluid thrill by placing the palm of your left hand flat on the left side of the child's abdomen and flicking the finger of your right hand on the right side of the abdomen; the movement of the fluid may be felt by your left hand.
- Repeat the procedure after asking the child (or the parent) to place the ulnar aspect of his/her hand longitudinally and firmly on the midline of the abdomen to prevent the transmission of the impulse through the subcutaneous fat of the abdominal wall. If you still feel the impulse, a massive amount of ascitic fluid is present.

4.11.3 Further Examination

To complete the abdominal examination, examine the following:

- **Groin**
  - Note any evidence of an inguinal hernia.
  - Inspect the diaper area for diaper rash.
- **Genitalia**
  - Examine the external genitalia of the child, if indicated.
  - Note any scrotal swelling. Testicular torsion may present as abdominal pain.
- **The posterior aspect of abdomen**
  - If the child is old enough, ask him/her to sit.
  - Inspect the back, looking for any deformities, swellings, scars, or any signs of spina bifida, which may cause constipation.
  - Palpate for sacral edema.
  - Palpate for tenderness over the vertebrae.
  - Check for renal angle tenderness by using the heel of your closed fist to strike the child gently over the renal angle.
  - If renal artery stenosis is suspected, listen carefully for renal bruits at the renal angles.
- **Anus**
  - Examine the anus, if relevant, guided by the clinical history of the child (e.g., inflammatory bowel disease).
  - Look for the position of the anus, patency, anal fissures, skin tags, fistulae, or excoriation.

- **Rectum**
  - The examination of the rectum is not routinely performed unless indicated. If it is needed, leave it until last. Before the examination explain what you are going to do, why it is necessary, and obtain consent.
  - The knee–chest position is preferred in infants and younger children, while older children are better examined in the left lateral position.
  - Carefully inspect the perianal skin for any lesions.
  - Look for any rectal prolapse.
  - Perform the examination using your little finger; it should be well lubricated and gloved.
  - Assess anal sphincter folds, anal tone, and the presence or absence of stool in the rectal ampulla.
- **Lower extremities**
  - Erythema nodosum: Bluish-red, tender, poorly defined nodules, 1–3 cm in diameter, often occurring over the extensor aspect of the legs. It may be a sign of systemic diseases, such as inflammatory bowel disease.
  - Inspect the toes for clubbing and note any koilonychia or leukonychia.

4.12 Examination of the Child's Genitalia

- Children are usually shy and reticent regarding genital examination. Therefore, it is very important to introduce yourself and to tell them clearly what you are going to do and why you need to do it. Furthermore, examination of the child's genitalia should not be performed unless a parent or a chaperone is present. You should record that in the visit notes [4].
- The technique of the examination of the child's genitalia must be tailored to his/her age.

Examination Station 4.6: Examination of the Child's Genitalia

1. **Male Genital Examination**
   - **Inspection**
     - Penis: size, position of the external urethral meatus, abnormalities (e.g., hypo–/epispadias)
     - Testes: descended or not
     - Scrotum: rugosities, swelling
   - **Palpation**
     - Groin: swelling (e.g., hernia, lymph node, or testis)
     - Scrotum: swellings (e.g., hydrocele, inguinal hernia, or enlarged testis)
     - Testes: descent of the testes in the scrotum, size of the testes

Continued on the next page

- **Special tests**
  - Transillumination test
2. **Female Genital Examination**
   - Clitoris: size and color
   - Labia majora: size, color, lesions, bruises, or rashes
   - Labia minora: abrasion, bruising, or scarring
   - Hymen: configuration and congenital variations
   - Urethral orifice: position and color

4.12.1 Male Genital Examination

- **Inspection**
- Inspect the genitalia while the child is in a standing or supine position, noting normality or deviation therefrom of the male external genitalia.
  - **Penis**
    Observe the penile size. A large penis may result from certain endocrine abnormalities, such as congenital adrenal hyperplasia. Micropenis is rare and usually an overdiagnosis.

    Look for circumcision and note any signs of inflammation of the glans penis (balanitis).

    Look for signs that suggest infection (e.g., penile discharge) or injury (e.g., bruising, abrasions, or scars).

    In children <u>older than 2 years</u>, retract the foreskin enough to see the external urethral meatus.

    Inspect the position of the external urethral meatus; normally it is positioned on the tip of the penis. In hypospadias, it is sited on the ventral surface of the penis, while in epispadias, it is sited on the dorsum of the penis [20].

    Examine the shaft of the penis, looking for any abnormalities.
  - **Scrotum and testes**
    Examine the child in a supine position and then in a standing position, if the child is old enough.

    Inspect the scrotum, looking for rugae.

    An underdeveloped scrotum may suggest undescended testes.

    Look for any groin or scrotal swelling. A swelling in the groin may suggest an enlarged lymph node, a hernia, or a testis. An enlarged scrotum may suggest a hydrocele, an inguinal hernia, or an enlarged testis.

    Note the change in the size of swelling while the child is crying or coughing.
- **Palpation**
  - Start palpation from the external inguinal ring and move downward toward the scrotum.
  - Palpate the testes gently with a warm hand, and, if possible, measure their size, using an orchidometer. Testicular size may be increased as in fragile X syndrome or decreased as in Klinefelter syndrome.

– The inability to feel the testis may suggest a retracted or undescended testis.
– A retracted testis can be gently milked down from the inguinal canal into the scrotum. If this is unsuccessful, repeat the procedure while the child is squatting or sitting cross-legged; this may be helpful. If not, the testes may be undescended (see Box 4.8) or absent.

Box 4.8: Cryptorchidism or Undescended Testis (UDT)

- Cryptorchidism is the failure of descent of one or both testes into the scrotum.
- It is very important to identify and treat cryptorchidism, because it may lead to infertility, testicular malignancy, or torsion [7].
- At birth, undescended testis occurs in about 3–4.5% of full-term male newborns and in up to 30% of preterm male newborns. Testes may continue to complete their descent until 4–6 months of age (the majority descend within the first 3 months of age).
- Failure of testicular descent by the age of 6 months requires referral to a surgical specialist for timely evaluation. Surgery should be performed by 9–15 months of age.

– If you find a scrotal swelling, palpate it for any tenderness (suggests torsion, infection, or trauma), and note whether it transilluminates [20].

You can differentiate a hydrocele from a hernia by the following:

– The cough impulse may be positive in the case of a hernia.
– You cannot get above the hernia by palpation.
– The testes cannot be palpated through the fluid if there is a hydrocele.
– Perform a transillumination test by placing the bright end of a flashlight (or a penlight) against the scrotal swelling. The scrotum will glow bright red in the case of a hydrocele [37].

4.12.2 Female Genital Examination

- In the presence of a parent or a female chaperone, place the female child in the supine position, and inspect the different structures of her genitalia, noting whether it is well-formed, and observing the presence and distribution of the pubic hair (may appears as early as 8 years of age, spreads downward in a triangular pattern, and points toward the vagina).
- Look for any abnormalities, such as a vaginal discharge, bleeding, and signs of sexual abuse or trauma, and consider the possibility of the presence of a foreign body, especially if there is a foul-smelling vaginal discharge.
- Do not palpate the female genitalia unless there is an indication (e.g., vaginal discharge, suspected sexual abuse, or foreign body).

Clitoris
- Inspect its size and color. Clitoris enlargement or pigmentation suggests congenital adrenal hyperplasia.

Labia Majora
- Inspect their size and color, and look for any lesions, bruises, or rashes.
- Note any labial fusion.

Labia Minora, Hymen, and Urethral Orifice
- Use both of your thumbs and gently separate the labia majora at their midpoint.
- Inspect the labia minora for any abnormalities suggesting trauma (e.g., abrasion, bruising, or scarring) or infection (e.g., discharge and malodor).
- Carefully inspect the hymenal orifice, noting its configuration, congenital variations, and patency.
- Look at the urethral orifice, noting its color and position. Normally, it is pink in color and located anterior to the vaginal orifice and posterior to the clitoris.

4.13   Reticuloendothelial System Examination

- The reticuloendothelial system consists of primary lymphoid organs (the bone marrow and thymus) and secondary lymphoid organs, such as the lymph nodes, tonsils, and spleen. The Kupffer cells of the liver are also part of this system.

Examination Station 4.7: Reticuloendothelial System Examination

Inspection
- **General inspection**
  - Level of consciousness
  - Nutritional status of the child
  - Skin rashes
  - Bruising or petechiae
  - Signs of respiratory distress
  - Visible lymphadenopathy
- **Face**
  - Jaundice
  - Pallor
  - Overgrowth of maxillary and frontal bones
- **Mouth**
  - Angular stomatitis or glossitis
  - Gum hypertrophy
  - Mucosal bleeding

Continued on the next page

- **Abdomen**
  - Distension
  - Dilated superficial veins
  - Scars

Palpation
- **Palpate for:**
  - The cervical lymph nodes
  - The axillary lymph nodes
  - The epitrochlear lymph nodes
  - The inguinal lymph nodes
  - The popliteal lymph nodes
- **Examine for hepatosplenomegaly.**
- **Take the temperature.**

Auscultation
- **Flow murmur, tachycardia**

Inspection
- **General inspection**
  - **Level of consciousness:** Look for lethargy or listlessness.
  - **Nutritional status of the child:** A child with reticuloendothelial system dysfunction may present with nonspecific signs or symptoms, such as weight loss.
  - **Skin rashes** may indicate an infection.
  - **Bruising or petechiae:** These may suggest thrombocytopenia, as in cases of leukemia or hypersplenism.
  - **Signs of respiratory distress** may suggest a respiratory tract infection [4].
  - **Visible lymphadenopathy:** Inspect the neck, axillae, and groin for visible lymphadenopathy (see Box 4.9).

Box 4.9: Lymphadenopathy

- Lymphadenopathy means enlargement of the lymph nodes, whether inflammatory or noninflammatory.
- Generalized lymphadenopathy can be defined as enlargement of the lymph nodes of three or more noncontiguous lymph node areas [13].

- **Face**
  - **Jaundice:** Inspect both sclerae for jaundice, which may be due to hepatobiliary diseases or hemolytic anemia.
  - **Pallor** suggests anemia.
  - **Overgrowth of maxillary and frontal bones** may point to bone marrow hyperplasia.

- **Mouth**
  - **Angular stomatitis and glossitis** may suggest riboflavin deficiency and anemia, respectively.
  - **Gum hypertrophy** may indicate leukemia.
  - **Mucosal bleeding** may suggest thrombocytopenia, which may occur in the case of hypersplenism [20].
- **Abdomen**
  - **Distension** may indicate organomegaly.
  - **Dilated superficial veins** may suggest portal hypertension.
  - **Scars:** Look for splenectomy scar.

Palpation

Palpate the lymph nodes symmetrically, from above downward.

- **Palpation of the cervical lymph nodes**
  - Place the child in the sitting position, and palpate the lymph nodes in both the anterior and the posterior triangles.
  - Begin the palpation by standing in front of the child and feeling the pre- and postauricular and the occipital nodes, as well the posterior triangles of the neck, using the pads of your second and third fingers.
  - Then stand behind the child, bend his/her head forward, and use both of your hands to palpate the submental, submandibular, tonsillar, supraclavicular, as well as the deep cervical lymph nodes (see Fig. 4.18).
- **Palpation of the axillary lymph nodes**
  - Palpate the axillary lymph nodes while the child is facing you in a sitting position (except for the subscapular group, which should be examined from behind).
  - Palpate the left axilla with your right hand and vice versa (except for the brachial group).
  - Use your fingertips to palpate the central, apical, pectoral, brachial, and subscapular groups of lymph nodes in turn (see below).

Central Group

  - Place your hand in the child's axilla while his/her arm is abducted; your palm should be directed toward the chest wall.
  - Ask the child to adduct his/her arm, resting it on your forearm.
  - Your other hand should be placed on the opposite shoulder of the child.
  - Palpate the central group with your fingers.

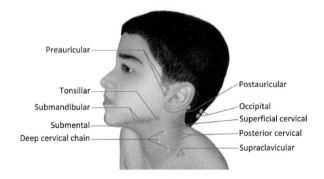

Fig. 4.18 Different groups of cervical lymph nodes. © Anwar Qais Saadoon

Apical Group
- Apply the same steps, but push your fingers into the axilla as high as possible.

Pectoral Group
- Palpate for this group of lymph nodes under the anterior axillary fold, using your thumb and fingers.

Brachial Group
- Palpate for this group of lymph nodes against the upper part of the humerus.
- Your palm should be directed laterally.
- Use your left hand to palpate the left side and your right hand to palpate the right side.

Subscapular Group
- Palpate for this group from behind.
- It is located on the posterior axillary fold.

- **Palpation of epitrochlear lymph nodes**
  - Support the child's wrist with your opposite hand; partially flex his/her elbow and supinate the forearm.
  - Use your thumb to palpate the epitrochlear lymph nodes in the anterior-medial region of the lower part of the arm.
- **Palpation of the inguinal lymph nodes**
  - Place the child in the supine position with thighs extended.
  - Gently palpate just below the inguinal ligament over the horizontal chain.
  - Then feel along the line of the saphenous vein for any enlarged node in the vertical chain.
- **Palpation of the popliteal lymph nodes**
  - Place the child in the supine position with knees flexed.
  - Palpate the popliteal fossa with the fingertips of both your hands.
- **Examine for hepatosplenomegaly** (see Sect. 4.11.2).
- **Take the temperature.**
  - Fever may indicate infection or may be due to other causes e.g., lymphoma and leukemia.

Clinical Tips 4.8

- If you find multiple enlarged lymph nodes, count their number and note the following for every single enlarged node:
  - Site
  - Size
  - Texture: hard, rubbery
  - Mobility
  - Warmth
  - Tenderness and erythema
- In addition, it is important to examine the areas of drainage, looking for any focus of infection.

Auscultation
- Auscultate the heart carefully. A flow murmur and tachycardia may indicate anemia.

4.14   Examination of the Nervous System

- Examination of the nervous system in children should be adapted according to the child's age.
- Take a careful birth history, concentrating on the perinatal period and antenatal disorders. Ask about Apgar scores, as they may provide clues to the current neurological disorder [1].
- Assess the developmental milestones of the young child (infant to 6 years), and get a good idea about maternal concerns. This is very important in evaluating mental status and cognition and crucial to the overall examination of the nervous system [2].

Examination Station 4.8: Examination of the Nervous System in Children

1. **General Physical Examination**
   - General observations
   - General appearance
   - Meningeal signs
   - Neck stiffness
   - Kernig sign
   - Brudzinski sign
2. **Mental Status Examination (MSE)**
3. **Cranial Nerve Examination**
4. **Motor System Examination**
   - Muscle bulk
   - Tone
   - Power
   - Involuntary movements
5. **Sensory System Examination**
   - Touch
   - Pain
   - Temperature
   - Proprioception
   - Vibration
   - Cortical localization

Continued on the next page

6. **Reflexes and Clonus**
   Reflexes
   - Superficial reflexes
   - Deep tendon reflexes
   - Primitive reflexes
   Clonus
7. **Coordination and Cerebellar Signs**
   - Speech
   - Tremor
   - Nystagmus
   - Nose–finger test
   - Dysdiadokokinesis
   - Heel–shin test
   - Gait

4.14.1 General Physical Examination

- **General observations**
  - Observe the presence of the following objects:
  Glasses
  Hearing aids
  Nasogastric or gastrostomy tubes
  Wheelchair
  Splints supporting the child's ankles, as in the case of hypertonia
  Diapers in older children
  - These may provide clues for underlying neurological disease [42].
- **General appearance**
  Top to toe
  - The head:
  Note the child's head shape and measure its size.
    Microcephaly or macrocephaly may be associated with neurological diseases.
    Plagiocephaly (flattening and asymmetry of the skull): When you look at the head from above, it looks like a parallelogram. This can be a postural deformity seen in normal infants and will correct with time as the child becomes mobile. It is more prominent in hypotonic nonmobile infants.
    Brachycephaly (flattening of the occiput with a reduction in anteroposterior diameter) is classically seen in Down syndrome.
    The prominence of the occiput may occur in Dandy–Walker syndrome [5].
    Fontanels: Palpate the fontanels, determining their size, tension, and whether bulged, flat, or depressed. Delayed closure or bulging of the fontanels may

suggest many pathologic conditions, including neurologic disorders (see Chap. 3).

- The face: Dysmorphic features may point to a syndrome that may be associated with neurologic disabilities or disorders (e.g., Down syndrome may be associated with mental retardation).
- The eyes: Look for squint, hyper- or hypotelorism, cataract, inability of eye closure, and note the ability of the child to fix his/her gaze on objects or people's faces.
- The ears: Note the position of the ears and any ear tags or skin lesions.
- The mouth: Look for mouth deviation, drooling, gum hypertrophy, and inspect the tongue, and teeth.
- The neck: Note any tracheostomy, torticollis, webbing, shunt, or scar.
- The back: Examine the back, looking for any sign of spinal dysraphism, such as sacral dimples and tufts of hair.
  - Skin/neurocutaneous lesions:
    Ash-leaf spots or hypopigmented patches, adenoma sebaceum, and Shagreen patches suggest tuberous sclerosis.
    Café au lait spots, and axillary and inguinal freckling, point to neurofibromatosis type I.
    Port-wine stain may suggest Sturge–Weber syndrome.
- Observe the child's posture, whether hemiplegic, scissoring (as in cerebral diplegia), or frog-like posture, which can be seen in the case of hypotonia.
  - Note any evidence of contractures.
- Observe the child's gait, if he/she is ambulant, noting different types of gaits (e.g., spastic, hemiparetic, steppage (as in sensory ataxia), and waddling gait (in myopathy)).
- **Meningeal signs**
  Examine for meningeal signs, when they are indicated.
  - **Neck stiffness**
    While the child is in the supine position, place your hand behind his/her head and try to flex the neck gently, or you can simply ask the conscious child to flex his/her neck and touch his/her chin to his/her chest.
    Undue resistance suggests meningeal irritation [13].
    Children under 2 years of age may not develop neck stiffness with meningitis.
  - **Kernig sign** (see Fig. 4.19a)
    Place the child in the supine position and flex his/her knee and hip on one side.
    While the hip is still flexed, gently extend the knee.
    Posterior thigh muscle pain and difficulty in knee extension are suggestive of meningeal irritation.
  - **Brudzinski sign** (see Fig. 4.19b)
    With the child supine, place your hand behind his/her head and the other hand on his/her chest to prevent him/her from rising while you are trying to flex his/her neck gently.
    Flexion of the knees and hips indicates a positive sign, which suggests meningeal irritation [13].

Fig. 4.19 Meningeal
signs: (**a**) Kernig sign and
(**b**) Brudzinski sign

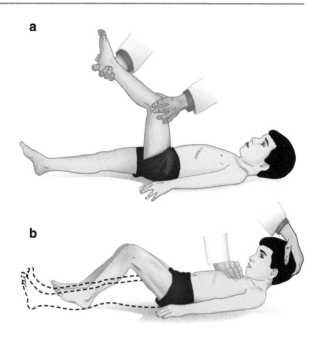

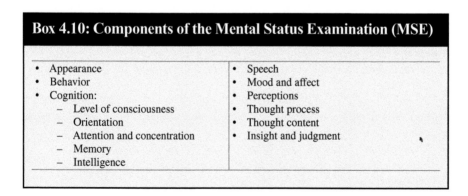

4.14.2   Mental Status Examination (MSE)

- Observations of the older child's play and having him/her complete a puzzle, tell
  a story, write a sentence, or draw a picture may give an idea about his/her mental
  status.
- If a formal examination of mental status is indicated, you should consider the
  different components of mental status examination (see Box 4.10).

Box 4.10: Components of the Mental Status Examination (MSE)

• Appearance	• Speech
• Behavior	• Mood and affect
• Cognition:	• Perceptions
– Level of consciousness	• Thought process
– Orientation	• Thought content
– Attention and concentration	• Insight and judgment
– Memory	
– Intelligence	

This section is not intended to be a comprehensive guide to the mental status examination. Examination of selective elements will be discussed here.

Level of Consciousness

- Many terms have been used to describe the state of consciousness (see Box 4.11).
- The Glasgow Coma Scale has been adapted to assess the level of consciousness for children; in this scoring system, three areas of brain function should be considered: speech (4 scores), eye opining (5 scores), and motor response (6 scores). The maximum score is 15, score ≤ 8 is serious, and the patient should be admitted to the ICU.

Box 4.11: Terminology of Altered States of Consciousness [35, 43]

- **Confusion:** The child has reduced awareness, disorientation, and bewilderment, as well as difficulty following commands. It can be a part of delirium.
- **Delirium:** The child is disoriented and unable to connect ideas and may have agitation, fearfulness, irritability, or even hallucination.
- **Lethargy:** The child has attention deficit and reduced wakefulness; he/she can be aroused by moderate stimuli, but then he/she returns to a sleep state again.
- **Obtundation:** This is similar to lethargy, but the child is drowsier even between the sleep states and has a slower response to stimuli and less interest in the environment.
- **Stupor:** The child can only be aroused by repeated, vigorous, and painful stimuli.
- **Coma:** The child is completely unarousable and unresponsive.

Orientation

- If the child is old enough, check for orientation by asking the child about the current time, place (ask him/her where he/she is now), and person (ask him/her to identify familiar people).

Attention

- A child who has inattention has difficulty concentrating on tasks or complex activities.
- To assess the child's attention, ask him/her to repeat a short list of items or numbers. The inability to repeat six or more items correctly may indicate attention deficit.
- This test can be affected by poor memory or by learning disabilities.
- You can also test the child's attention by asking him/her to spell a word backward.

Speech and Language Function

- Listen to the child's spontaneous speech, noting the articulation of words, fluency, rate, tone, and volume of the speech.
- Note any abnormal language (e.g., neologisms).

Key Points 4.3

- Influent speech may suggest damage in Broca's area, which causes expressive (motor) dysphasia.
- **Dysphasia** is disturbance of language function (speech production and/or understanding); it usually occurs due to dominant cerebral hemisphere lesions. It should be differentiated from **dysphonia** (impairment in the voice volume, quality, or pitch due to vagus nerve palsy or laryngeal diseases or injury) and **dysarthria** (difficulty in articulation or resonation due to muscle diseases or cranial nerves palsies).

4.14.3 Cranial Nerves Examination

4.14.3.1   CN I (Olfactory Nerve)
- It is not routinely examined unless indicated.
- Ask the child if he/she has a sense of smell and whether he/she has noticed any changes.
- Ensure that both nostrils are open.
- Ask the child to close his/her eyes.
- Close one nostril at a time.
- Test the smell sense using common nonirritant odors (e.g., chocolate, coffee, or orange peel).
- Ask the child to say "yes" when he/she smells a new odor [37].

4.14.3.2   CN II (Optic Nerve)
Examination of the optic nerve includes visual acuity, pupils, visual field, and fundoscopy.

1. **Visual acuity**
   - Many charts can be used to test visual acuity according to the child's age. For example, Cardiff acuity cards (7 months–3 years), tumbling E (3–5 years), and Snellen charts (in children older than 5 years) [20].
   - Test each eye individually while covering up the other one.
   - Visual acuity is difficult to assess in young children, but it can be roughly tested by checking the ability of the infant to fix and follow a silent moving object. Generally, <u>babies should fix and follow objects by age 6–8 weeks</u> [42].
2. **Pupils**
   Inspect the pupils; they should be round and symmetrical on both sides.
   - **Red reflex**
     – In a slightly darkened room, use an ophthalmoscope (holding it 20 cm–30 cm away, with a +4 convex lens) to shine light through the pupils of both eyes, looking for the red reflex of each pupil.

- The absence of a red reflex or the presence of a white reflex may suggest serious conditions (e.g., cataract, retinoblastoma, or retinal detachment) [37, 42].
- **Pupillary reflex:** Test both eyes for pupillary reflex by shining light from the side into one eye while the other is shielded, and notice the pupil responses, looking for any abnormalities (see Box 4.12):
  - Direct light reflex: pupillary constriction on the same (stimulated) eye
  - Consensual light reflex: pupillary constriction on the other eye

---

Box 4.12: Relative Afferent Pupillary Defect (RAPD)

- When you shine light into the eye, it will be transmitted by the optic nerve (the afferent pathway). As a result, the pupil of the same eye constricts via the parasympathetic branch within the oculomotor nerve (the efferent pathway), and the pupil of the other eye also constricts due to activation of the efferent pathway on the opposite side (the consensual light reflex).
- In dim light, note the pupils size and perform **swinging flashlight test** with the child fixing on a distant target by directing a bright focal light alternately into each eye in turn.
- Swinging the light to the unaffected eye leads to pupillary constriction in both eyes. Swinging the light back to the affected eye leads to partial dilation of both pupils. This responce is **a relative afferent pupillary defect (RAPD).**
- Relative afferent pupillary defect (RAPD) suggests optic nerve diseases [42].

- **Accommodation**
  - Ask the child to look at the ceiling.
  - Hold your finger close to his/her nose and ask him/her to focus on it.
  - The typical response is convergence of the eyes and constriction of the pupils.

3. **Visual fields**
   - Examine the visual fields by confrontation.
   - Sit 1 m away from the child.
   - Your eyes should be at the same level as the child's eyes.
   - Explain clearly what you would like him/her to do.
   - Ask the child to cover one eye and look directly into your opposite eye.
   - Shut your eye that is opposite the child's covered eye and bring an object from outside his/her field of vision.
   - Ask him/her to say "yes" when he/she sees the object.
   - Test one eye at a time with the other eye closed or covered.
   - Exclude sensory inattention by examining both eyes together.
   - Examine for central scotoma by holding a small red pin midway between yourself and the child and ask him/her to focus on your eye while he/she is closing one eye. Try to compare your visual field with that of the child.

- In a young child, visual fields can be tested by using two objects. Hold an interesting toy in the central field of the child's vision, and ask another examiner to bring a more interesting toy slowly into the peripheral fields of the child's vision from behind. Observe the movement of the child's gaze toward the second toy.

4. **Fundoscopy**
   - If indicated (e.g., absent red reflex), perform a fundoscopic examination at the end of the examination.
   - Pull the curtains and dim the room lights.
   - Explain to the child that you are going to look at his/her eyes.
   - Ask the child to focus on a distant point.
   - Hold the ophthalmoscope in your right hand, and approach the child's right eye from his/her right side, using your right eye.
   - From a distance of 20 cm, bring the red reflex into focus.
   - Then come close to the child's head, and adjust the lens until the retina comes into focus.
   - Examine the lens, disc, cup margins, vessels, and retinal surface, looking for abnormalities such as optic atrophy, papilledema, choroidoretinitis, cherry red spot, etc.
   - Repeat the same on the child's left eye, holding the ophthalmoscope in your left hand and using your left eye.

Notes 4.10

- Mydriatics are usually not needed in older children, but they are still required in infants.
- In young children, fundoscopic examination is difficult and an ophthalmological opinion may be required [37].

4.14.3.3 CN III (Oculomotor Nerve), CN IV (Trochlear Nerve), and CN VI (Abducens Nerve)

- Inspect the eyes, looking for any ptosis, nystagmus, or squint, excluding any nerves palsies (see Box 4.13).
- Inspect the size, shape, and symmetry of the pupils and their reaction to light (reflexes).
- Examine eye movements in the four cardinal directions, as follows:
  - Move your finger or an interesting toy around the field of view of the child.
  - Ask the child to follow your finger with his/her eyes, without moving his/her head.
  - You may need to hold the child's head still.
  - Extreme lateral gaze should be avoided, as it may result in nystagmus in normal children.
  - Note whether the eye movements are conjugate or not.
  - Ask the child to tell you if he/she can see two fingers at any point.

Box 4.13: Oculomotor, Trochlear, and Abducens Nerve Palsies

- III cranial nerve (oculomotor nerve) palsy results in dilatation of the pupil, associated with the absence of light reflexes, as well as ptosis and eye deviation downward and outward.
- IV cranial nerve (trochlear nerve) palsy leads to the inability to abduct the eye while looking downward.
- VI cranial nerve (abducens nerve) palsy causes a convergent squint and inability to abduct the eye [44].

4.14.3.4   CN V (Trigeminal Nerve)
- **Motor function**
  - Ask the child to open his/her mouth against resistance and to clench his/her teeth.
  - Palpate the masseter and temporal muscles while the teeth are clenched.
- **Sensory function**
  - With the child's eyes closed, check the sensation to light touch, pain, and temperature in areas that are supplied by the ophthalmic, maxillary, and mandibular divisions of the trigeminal nerve.
- **Corneal reflex**
  - The afferent limb of this reflex is the trigeminal nerve, and the efferent limb is the facial nerve [5].
  - Corneal reflex is not routinely tested in children. If it is indicated, ask the child to look upward and lightly touch the lateral edge of the cornea with a fine wisp of cotton. See whether or not the child blinks [13, 20].

4.14.3.5   CN VII (Facial Nerve)
Inspect the child's face at rest, looking for asymmetry and noting the palpebral fissures, eye closure, nasolabial folds, and the mouth angles.

- **Motor function**
  Ask the child to:
  - Squeeze his/her eyes closed as tightly as possible
  - Raise his/her eyebrows
  - Smile and show his/her teeth
  - Puff out his/her cheeks
- **Sensory function**
  - If indicated, check the child's taste over the anterior two-thirds of the tongue, using natural tastes (e.g., lemon juice, sugar, or salt).
- **Corneal reflex**
  - Corneal reflex is not routinely tested in children unless indicated (see above).

4.14.3.6   CN VIII (Vestibulocochlear Nerve)

1. **Cochlear**
   - Inspect the external auditory meatus, looking for any local disease, wax, or abnormalities.
   - Ask about speech and hearing. If there is any concern, you may do a hearing test.
   - Listen to the child's speech to ascertain whether it is normal or not.
   - In a young child who is lying down, you can ring a bell and see whether he/she turns his/her head toward the sound.
   - In children older than 4 years, test hearing by whispering numbers in each ear while masking hearing in the other ear by rubbing the tragus, and ask the child to repeat them.
   - If there is deafness, differentiate whether it is sensory neural or conductive hearing loss by Weber and Rinne tests [44].
   - **Weber Test**
     The Weber test can be performed in an older child by applying a vibrating tuning fork (256 or 512 Hz) to the center of the child's frontal bone or to the incisors, asking him/her if he/she hears the sound louder in one ear than in the other.
     A healthy child should hear the sound equally loud in both ears (no lateralization).
     In the case of sensory neural hearing loss, the sound will be louder on the healthy side.
     In conductive hearing loss, the sound will be louder on the diseased side.
     The Weber test is not useful in the diagnosis of symmetrical hearing loss [3, 37].
   - **Rinne Test**
     The Rinne test can be performed in children older than 6 years of age.
     Place a vibrating tuning fork (256 or 512 Hz) just in front of the ear, without touching (testing the air conduction). Then place the base of a still-vibrating tuning fork on the mastoid process behind the ear (testing the bone conduction).
     Ask the child where the sound is louder, in front or behind the ear.
     Normally, the conduction of the air is better than that of the bone (positive Rinne).
     In conductive hearing loss, the bone conduction is louder (negative Rinne) [13].
     In the case of sensory neural hearing loss, air conduction is louder or equal to that of the bone conduction.

2. **Vestibular**
   - Check for balance of gait and examine for nystagmus.

4.14.3.7   CN IX (Glossopharyngeal Nerve) and CN X (Vagus Nerve)

- Listen to the child's voice for any dysphonia or difficulty in speech.
- Ask the child to say "ah," and watch the movements of the palate and uvula, looking for any abnormalities, such as deviation of the uvula.
- Ask the child to cough.
- Examine the swallowing of the child by asking him/her to swallow a sip of water.
- Test for the taste sensation in the posterior third of the tongue (if indicated).
- Use an orange stick to gently test sensation on both sides of the pharynx (if indicated, in children with swallowing difficulties).
- Do not examine the gag reflex in children unless indicated [13].

4.14.3.8   CN XI (Accessory Nerve)

- Face the child, noting any wasting or hypertrophy of the sternocleidomastoid muscles and palpate them to assess their bulk, then inspect the trapezius musles while you are standing behind the child, noting any wasting or asymmetry.
- Examine the power of the sternocleidomastoid muscles by asking the child to turn his/her head to the side while you are resisting its movement with your hand.
- Then assess the trapezius muscle by asking the child to shrug his/her shoulders.

4.14.3.9   CN XII (Hypoglossal Nerve)

- Ask the child to stick out his/her tongue and move it from side to side.
- Note whether there is any atrophy, fasciculation, or deviation of the tongue.
- Then ask the child to push his/her tongue against the inside of each cheek while you assess the power of the tongue muscle from the outside.

4.14.4 Motor System Examination

- **Muscle bulk**
  - Decreased muscle bulk (atrophy) can occur due to lower motor neuron lesions or disuse atrophy.
  - Increased muscle bulk (hypertrophy) is typically physiologic (e.g., bodybuilders).
  - Bilateral calf hypertrophy associated with weakness "pseudohypertrophy" (due to replacement of the muscle by fat and connective tissue) may suggest Duchenne muscular dystrophy [37].
- **Tone**
  - Tone can be defined as muscle resistance against passive stretch. The child may have normal tone; decreased muscle tone (hypotonia), e.g., a lower motor neuron lesion; or increased muscle tone (hypertonia/spasticity/rigidity), e.g., an upper motor neuron lesion.
  - With the child supine, passively flex and extend his/her main joints in their range of movement, feeling for resistance and comparing side by side [42].

In infants, tone can be assessed by the following:

Posture
- This can provide a clue about the tone (e.g., a frog-like posture of the legs suggests hypotonia, which may occur in the case of a lower motor neuron lesion).

Traction Response (Pull to Sit)
- Grasp the infant's hands and gently pull him/her from the supine to the sitting position while you are watching his/her head. In infants aged 4 months or more, the head should be brought up rapidly to a position in line with the trunk. In the case of hypotonia, the head lags backward, and when an erect position is assumed, it drops forward, while in hypertonia, the infant's head is maintained backwards [35].

Axillary (Vertical) Suspension
- Hold the infant's chest with your hands and suspend the baby, lifting him/her in an upright position while you are watching his/her legs.
- A hypotonic infant tends to slip through your hands.
- In the case of cerebral palsy or other causes of spasticity, you will see scissoring or hyperextension of the legs [37].

Ventral (Horizontal) Suspension
- With the infant prone, put your hand under his/her trunk, and gently lift the infant upward.
- Generally, by the age of 3–12 months, he/she brings his/her head above the level of his/her back, and the back is slightly extended.
- A hypotonic infant will droop over your hands like a rag doll [35].

- **Power (muscle strength)**
    - Observation of a child's crawling, walking, running, hopping, jumping, climbing steps, or squatting can provide a hint about his/her muscle power.
    - In an old-enough, cooperative child, assess the grade of the power in various groups of limb muscles according to the following scale:
      Grade 0— no movement (no contraction)
      Grade 1—minimal movement present (visible or palpable flicker or trace of contraction)
      Grade 2—active movement, but not against gravity
      Grade 3—active movement against gravity, but not against resistance
      Grade 4—active movement against gravity along with some externally applied resistance (less than normal)
      Grade 5—active movement against gravity along with good externally applied resistance (normal power)
    - Note the symmetry of active movement while assessing the power, comparing side by side.
    - If the child is old enough, assess whether he/she has the ability to stand up from a prone position. If the child uses his/her hands to climb up his/her legs to compensate for weakness of the proximal muscles in the lower limbs, this

is known as "**Gower sign**," which is a classic sign of Duchenne muscular dystrophy [37].
- **Involuntary movements**
  - Note any fasciculation (a brief, involuntary contraction and relaxation affecting a small number of muscle fibers). Although fasciculation can be seen in normal children, it may indicate a lower motor neuron lesion, as in motor neuron disease.
  - Look for any abnormal movements—e.g., chorea (brief, purposeless, irregular, and involuntary movements commonly affecting the face or the arms) or athetosis (writhing, involuntary movements, slower than chorea, usually affecting the proximal limbs).

4.14.5 Sensory System Examination

- Testing of the sensory modalities includes the following: touch, pain, temperature, vibration, and joint position (proprioception), in addition to cortical localization.
- You should ask the child to close his/her eyes while you are testing his/her sensation.

Touch
- Assess light touch by stimulating the skin using a wisp of cotton wool [27].
- Ask the child to close his/her eyes and to say "yes" directly when he/she feels the cotton wool touch his/her skin.
- You should touch the child's skin at each of these sites:
  - Lateral surface of the upper arm (C5)
  - Tip of the thumb (C6)
  - The web between the index and middle fingers (C7)
  - Tip of the little finger (C8)
  - Medial surface of the lower arm (T1)
  - Medial surface of the upper arm (T2)
- Test for sharp touch using a blunt hatpin or an orange stick.

Pain
- Test for the pain sensation using a new pin.

Temperature
- Immerse a metal object (such as a tuning fork) in cold and warm water, and use it to test for temperature. (You can also use a cold spray or warm hands for testing.)

Joint position (proprioception)
- Hold the middle phalanx of the child's index finger with your index finger and thumb, and grasp the distal phalanx by the sides with the index finger and thumb of your other hand, then move it up and down.
- Tell the child what you mean by "up" and "down."

- Ask the child to close his/her eyes.
- Then repeat the test, moving the distal phalanx three to four times and resting either at the up or the down point.
- Ask the child to tell you the position of the distal phalanx, whether up or down.
- Repeat the test for different positions.

Vibration
- This is hard to test in children.
- Using a 128 Hz tuning fork, check for vibration.
- Apply the tuning fork to the distal phalanx of the big toe, just below the nail bed.
- Place your finger on the other side of the joint being tested, to compare the child's threshold of vibration perception with your own.

Cortical Localization
Cortical localization includes:
- Two-point discrimination
- Astereognosis (the child is unable to identify objects placed in his/her hands based on touch alone in the absence of other sensory inputs)
- Graphesthesia (the child's ability to identify letters or numbers that are drawn onto his/her palm purely by the sensation of touch)
- Point localization
- Sensory inattention

4.14.6 Reflexes and Clonus

4.14.6.1 Reflexes
Examine for superficial and deep reflexes.

- **Superficial reflexes**
  - Abdominal wall reflex (T7 to T12)
    Stroke the abdominal wall from the lateral to the medial side.
    Look for contraction of the anterior abdominal wall muscles.
  - Cremasteric reflex (L1)
    Stroke a line along the medial thigh to elicit this reflex, looking for the movement of the testis.
    Normally, there will be elevation of the ipsilateral testis.
  - Plantar response (S1, S2)
    Firmly stroke the lateral border of the sole of the child's foot, using your thumbnail or a blunt, pointed object.
    The test is negative when there is a plantar flexion of the big toe.
    A dorsiflexion of the big toe is considered positive (positive Babinski sign) and is suggestive of an upper motor neuron lesion [13].
- **Deep tendon reflexes**
  - Elicitation of the tendon reflex should be left until last.
  - Explain what you are going to do.

- While the child is relaxing and his/her head is central, elicit each reflex by stroking the tendon with a tendon hammer and watching the contraction and relaxation of the muscle that is expected to contract, comparing each reflex with the other side.
  Biceps reflex C5 (C6)
  Triceps reflex C7 (C8)
  Supinator (brachioradialis) reflex C5 (C6)
  Knee reflex (L2), L3, L4
  Ankle reflex S1
- The reflex may be absent (suggests a neuromuscular problem, a lesion within the spinal cord, or poor examination technique), sluggish, or present only with reinforcement, readily elicited, brisk (as in anxiety or a pyramidal disorder) without clonus or associated with clonus.
- **Reinforcement of reflexes**
  - Before concluding that a reflex is absent, try to reinforce the finding by asking the child to clench his/her teeth tightly or to hook his/her hands together and pull them apart strenuously, immediately before you strike the tendon.
- **Primitive reflexes**
  - Elicit primitive reflexes in infants (see Chap. 3, Table 3.4).

4.14.6.2   Clonus
- Carry out a sharp dorsiflexion to the relaxed child's ankle while you are grasping it.
- Rhythmic jerking movements (more than three beats) are called "clonus." This may be felt or seen in the muscles of the calf in cases of hypertonia.

4.14.7 Coordination and Cerebellar Signs

- **Speech**
  - Carefully listen to the speech of the child, noting its quality.
  - Slurred speech may suggest a cerebellar lesion [13].
- **Nystagmus**
  - Ask the child to look at your finger while you are moving it to the sides, as well as up and down
  - Observe the movements of the child's eyes. An involuntary, rhythmic, jerking movement of the eye is called "nystagmus." It may be a sign of cerebellar disease or visual impairment [42].
- **Tremor**
  - Intention tremor may occur on reaching for an object.
  - The finger–nose test is a test for intention tremor. It can be performed by asking the child to touch the tip of his/her nose with his/her index finger and then to reach out and touch the tip of your finger. Ask the child to repeat the maneuver as quickly as possible while you are moving your finger. The presence of tremors at the time when the finger of the child begins approaching the target suggests cerebellar disease.
  - Oscillation of outstretched arms also may indicate cerebellar disease.

Fig. 4.20 The
heel–shin test

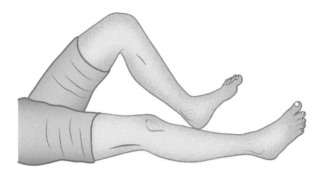

- **Heel–shin test** (see Fig. 4.20)
  - With the child supine, ask him/her to slide the heel of his/her foot down the front of the shin of the opposite leg and to repeat the maneuver several times, as quickly as possible.
  - Note how accurately this is performed by the child.
- **Dysdiadokokinesis**
  - Ask the child to quickly and repeatedly tap one hand with the other, alternating between front and back (rapid alternating movements).
  - The inability to perform this action is called dysdiadochokinesia.
- **Gait**
  - Observe the child's gait, looking for a wide-based gait, which suggests cerebellar ataxia.
  - Ask the child to walk a straight line, with one foot immediately in front the other (the toes of the back foot touching the heel of the front foot with each step. This is known as **tandem gait**). It highlights even subtle difficulties with balance.
- **Romberg's sign**
  - Test for this sign when there is evidence of ataxia.
  - Ask the child to stand with feet together and eyes open.
  - Watch the child for a few seconds. Then ask him/her to close his/her eyes, noting any unsteadiness that may result from loss of postural sensation.

4.15   Musculoskeletal System Examination

- Many musculoskeletal conditions can be diagnosed by history and examination alone.
- Neurologic assessment is an important part of examination of the musculoskeletal system in children.
- The child should be comfortable and adequately exposed.

- It is preferable to examine infants and young children on their parent's lap. In this way, you may get their cooperation. This position makes them feel more comfortable and secure [45].

Examination Station 4.9: Musculoskeletal System Examination

1. **General Physical Examination**
   - General observations
   - Posture
   - Gait
   - Extremities
   - Back and spine
   - Measurements
     - Limb circumference
     - Limb length
2. **Examination of the Joints**
   - **Inspection (look)**
     - Guarding
     - Swelling
     - Deformities and contractures
     - Skin changes: redness, rashes, bruising, sinuses, or scars
     - Changes of adjacent structure: muscle bulk (atrophy or hypertrophy)
   - **Palpation (feel)**
     - Swelling
     - Tenderness
     - Temperature
     - Crepitus
     - Fluid thrill
   - **Range of motion (move)**
     - Cervical spine
     - Temporomandibular joint
     - Shoulder joints
     - Thoracolumbar spine
     - Elbows
     - Radioulnar joints
     - Wrists
     - Metacarpophalangeal joints
     - Hips
     - Knees
     - Ankles
     - Feet

4.15.1 General Physical Examination

- **General observations**
  - In infants, notice crawling, bottom-shuffling, and how he/she reaches the objects.
  - Assess child's growth and nutritional status: Chronic musculoskeletal disorder may be associated with poor growth [42].
  - Skin: Skin diseases may be associated with musculoskeletal disorders, and vice versa. Inspect the child's skin, noting any lesion, e.g., psoriatic lesions, café au lait spots, dimples, hairy patches, cysts, tufts of hair. Skin rash can be a feature of systemic illness with joint involvement, e.g., SLE and rheumatoid arthritis.
  - Others: Wheelchairs, splints, crutches, bandages, plaster of Paris, and traction may all provide clues about the child's condition.
- **Posture**
  - The child's posture may offer a clue to the musculoskeletal problem (e.g., a child with a "pulled" elbow may hold his/her arm extended and internally rotated, parallel to his/her body).
- **Gait**
  - In general, children can start walking between 8 and 16 months of age [45].
  - Assess the child's gait, looking for the rhythm, symmetry of movements, and whether there is any limp.
  - A single gait cycle comprises two phases: stance (the foot is in contact with the ground) and swing (the foot swings forward without ground contact). Normal gait is smooth and symmetric.
  - Observation of the child's gait may offer clues about the functional effects of many disorders.
  - Abnormalities in gait can be seen in conditions that cause muscle weakness (such as spina bifida or muscular dystrophy), contractures (such as arthrogryposis), or spasticity (such as cerebral palsy).
- **Extremities**
  - Inspect the upper limbs, looking for any abnormalities and deformities.
  - Carefully inspect both hands, looking for deformities and muscle wasting. Count the number of fingers and look for any deformities, such as thumb clenching or incurving of the little finger.
  - Inspect the legs and feet, looking for any asymmetry, abnormalities, and deformities, such as talipes or bow legs, and count the number of toes.
- **Back and spine**
  - Inspect the back, looking for any deformities, such as scoliosis, kyphosis, or lordosis, and note any limitation in the back movements, spina bifida, pilonidal dimple, tufts of hair, sinuses, swelling, and Mongolian spots.
  - Examine for scoliosis
    With the child standing with feet together, inspect the back from behind, looking for apparent curving of the lumbar or thoracic spine to the right or left and asymmetry of the shoulders (the shoulder is elevated on the convex side).

Ask the child to bend forward to touch his/her toes, and inspect the back carefully from behind. Postural scoliosis (e.g., unequal leg length or unilateral muscle spasm secondary to pain) will disappear on bending, while fixed scoliosis will evidence by a gibbus or hump.

- **Measurements**
  - **Limb circumference**
    Use a non-stretchable tape to measure the circumference of the lower limbs from a set point above and below the tibial tuberosity (e.g., 10 cm above and 5 cm below), looking for any muscle wasting.
  - **Limb length**
    Ask the child to lie on a flat surface and use a non-stretchable tape to measure the true leg length from the anterior superior iliac spine to the medial malleolus, or apparent leg length from the pubic symphysis to the medial malleolus.

4.15.2 Examination of the Joints

- **Inspection**
  - **Guarding**
    The child may protect the affected area or joint with his/her hand, by limping, or by avoiding the use of that joint.
    This behavior may suggest a significant injury to the affected area or joint.
  - **Swelling**
    Joint swelling may suggest effusion, fracture, or a tumor.
    It may be subtle and difficult to discover. Therefore, comparison of both sides is required.
  - **Deformities and contracture**
    A deformity may offer a clue to an underlying fracture or other musculoskeletal problems.
    Contractures can be congenital (as in arthrogryposis) or acquired.
  - **Skin changes**
    Redness may suggest inflammation, infection, or injury.
    Bruising: The presence of bruising may indicate an underlying injury.
  - **Changes of adjacent structure**
    Muscle bulk: Look for muscle atrophy or hypertrophy.
- **Palpation**
  - **Swelling**
    If there is a swelling, palpate it, noting whether it is hard (bony), soft (suggests synovitis), or fluctuant as in joint effusion.
  - **Tenderness**: While you are palpating the affected area, look at the child's face, noting any grimacing or other signs of tenderness.
  - **Temperature**
    With the back of your hand, feel the joint for temperature, comparing both sides at the same time.
    The increased joint temperature may suggest an infection or a chronic joint inflammation.

- **Crepitus:** Feel for crepitus (can be felt as creaking or bubbling) while you are flexing and extending the joint. Its presence suggests a joint inflammation or degenerative changes.
- **Fluid thrill**: Examine the knee joints for effusion by doing the **bulge test** (see Fig. 4.21) and **patellar tap test** (see Fig. 4.22).
- **Palpation of the spine**: Run your fingers along the child's spine, excluding spinal defects and detecting the presence of tenderness or any masses.
- **Range of motion**

If the child is old enough, ask him/her to move his/her joints actively in all directions, as per the following:

- **Cervical spine**

  Flexion

  Extension

  Lateral rotation

  Lateral flexion

- **Temporomandibular joint**

  Ask the child to open his/her mouth as wide as possible, and feel for crepitus.

- **Shoulder joints**

  Abduction

  Adduction

  Flexion

  Extension

  Superior and inferior rotation

- **Thoracolumbar spine**

  Flexion

  Extension

  Rotation

  Lateral flexion

- **Elbows**

  Flexion

  Extension

- **Radioulnar joint**

  Pronation

  Supination

The elbow should be flexed and fixed to prevent shoulder movement.

- **Wrists**
  - Dorsiflexion (extension)
  - Palmar flexion (flexion)
- **Metacarpophalangeal joints**
  - Ask the child to move his/her fingers and to open and close his/her fists.
- **Hips**
  - Flexion
  - Extension and both internal and external rotation
  - Abduction
  - Adduction

The pelvis should be stabilized while you are moving the hip.

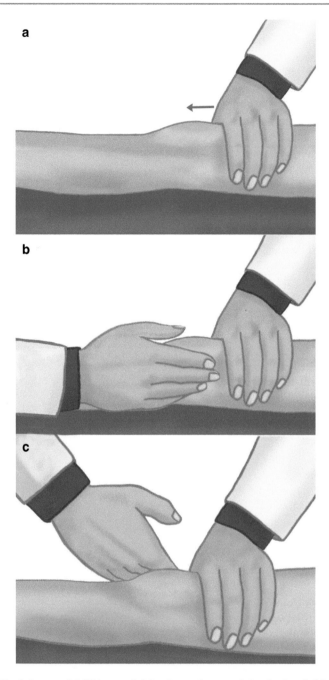

Fig. 4.21 The bulge test. (**a**) Slide your left hand over the extended and relaxed child's leg (start over the thigh, above the patella, until you reach the upper patellar edge), massaging the fluid down from the suprapatellar pouch, using the palm of your hand and maintaining the hand there. (**b**) Stroke the medial aspect of the joint, displacing excess fluid to the lateral side of the joint. (**c**) Then stroke the lateral side of the joint by your right hand and watch carefully for any bulge on the medial aspect of the joint. ©Anwar Qais Saadoon

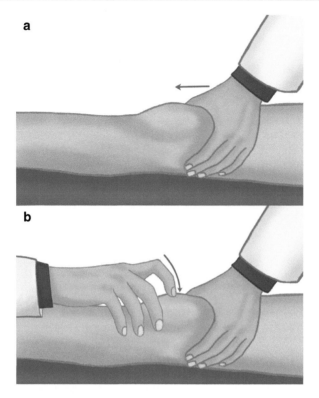

Fig. 4.22 The patellar tap test. (**a**) With the child's knee extended, empty the suprapatellar pouch of fluid with the palm of your left hand, as shown. (**b**) Press briskly and firmly over the patella with the index finger of your right hand. Palpate and observe for a "bouncing" mobility as the femur is struck by the patella. A patellar tap indicates increased fluid in the joint space. ©Anwar Qais Saadoon

- **Knees**
  - Flexion
  - Extension

Ankles (consist of three joints each)

- **Tibiotalar joint**
  - Dorsiflexion
  - Plantarflexion
- **Subtalar joint**
  - Inversion
  - Eversion
- **Midtarsal joints**
  - Medial and lateral movements of the forefoot.

- **Feet**
  - Inspect the arches.
  - Movements of the toes: flexion, extension, adduction, abduction, or circumduction.

    Note any limitation in movements, and observe the child's face for signs of pain.

    Passively move the joints in the range of movement, noting any evidence of pain and feeling for any resistance or crepitation, comparing side by side.

    Ask the child if it is painful somewhere.

    In younger children, observe the child's movements and actions. This can offer clues about the integrity of joint function.

References

1. Gill D, O'Brien N. Pediatric clinical examination made easy. 6th ed. Edinburgh: Elsevier; 2018.
2. Melman S. The physical examination. In: Zorc JJ, Alpern ER, Brown LW, Loomes KM, Marino BS, Mollen CJ, et al., editors. Schwartz's clinical handbook of pediatrics. 5th ed. Philadelphia: Lippincott Williams & Wilkins Business; 2013. p. 6–34.
3. Snadden D, Laing R, Potts S, Nicol F, Colledge N. History taking and general examination. In: Douglas G, Nicol F, Robertson C, editors. Macleod's clinical examination. 13th ed. Edinburgh: Elsevier; 2013. p. 1–63.
4. Gupte S, Smith R. Pediatric history-taking and clinical examination. In: Gupte S, editor. The short textbook of pediatrics. 12th ed. New Delhi: Jaypee Brothers Medical Publishers; 2016. p. 19–37.
5. Greenbaum LA. Deficit Therapy. In: Kleigman RM, Stanton BF, Schor NF, St Geme III JW, Behrman RE, editors. Nelson textbook of pediatrics. 20th ed. Philadelphia: Elsevier; 2016. p. 388–390.
6. Freedman S. Oral rehydration therapy. In: Mattoo TK, Stack AM, Kim MS, editors. UpToDate. 2017. http://www.uptodate.com/contents/oral-rehydration-therapy. Accessed 9 Feb 2018.
7. Booth IW, Jenkins H, Lander A, Whyte L, Puntis J. Gastroenterology. In: Lissauer T, Carroll W, editors. Illustrated textbook of pediatrics. 5th ed. Edinburgh: Elsevier; 2018. p. 234–55.
8. Stead LG, Stead SM, Kaufman MS. First aid for the pediatrics clerkship: a student to student guide. 2nd ed. Boston: McGraw-Hill; 2004.
9. World Health Organization, UNICEF. IMCI handbook: integrated management of childhood illness. Geneva: World Health Organization; 2005. http://www.who.int/maternal_child_adolescent/documents/9241546441/en/. Accessed 17 Dec 2017.
10. World Health Organization. Pocket book of hospital care for children: guidelines for the management of common childhood illnesses. 2nd ed. Geneva: World Health Organization; 2013. http://www.who.int/maternal_child_adolescent/documents/child_hospital_care/en/. Accessed 17 Dec 2017.
11. Goday PS. Malnutrition in children in resource-limited countries: clinical assessment. In: Motil KJ, Li BU, Hoppin AG, editors. UpToDate. 2017. http://www.uptodate.com/contents/malnutrition-in-children-in-resource-limited-countries-clinical-assessment?source=search_result&search=Malnutrition+in+developing+countries%3A+Clinical+assessment&selectedTitle=1%7E150. Accessed 9 Feb 2018.
12. World Health Organization, United Nations children's Fund. WHO child growth standards and the identification of severe acute malnutrition in infants and children. Geneva: World Health Organization; 2009. http://www.who.int/nutrition/publications/severemalnutrition/9789241598163/en/. Accessed 4 July 2018.

13. Narang M. Approach to practical pediatrics. 2nd ed. New Delhi: Jaypee Brothers Medical Publishers; 2011.
14. Mehta M. Malnutrition. In: Parthasarathy A, Gupta P, Nair M, Menon P, Agarwal RK, Sukumaran T, editors. IAP textbook of pediatrics. 5th ed. New Delhi: Jaypee Brothers Medical Publishers; 2013. p. 134–49.
15. Puntis JW. Clinical evaluation and anthropometry. In: Koletzko B, Bhatia J, Bhutta ZA, Cooper P, Makrides M, Uauy R, et al., editors. Pediatric nutrition in practice. World review of nutrition and dietetics, vol. 113. 2nd ed. Nestec: Basel; 2015. p. 6–14.
16. Sidwell RU, Thomson MA. Easy pediatrics. Boca Raton: CRC Press; 2011.
17. Kelnar CJ, Butler GE. Endocrine gland disorders and disorders of growth and puberty. In: Mcintosh N, Helms PJ, Smyth RL, Logan S, editors. Forfar and Arneil's textbook of pediatrics. 7th ed. Edinburgh: Elsevier; 2008. p. 409–512.
18. Centers for Disease Control and Prevention. WHO growth standards. 2009. https://www.cdc.gov/growthcharts/data/who/GrChrt_Boys_24HdCirc-L4W_rev90910.pdf. Accessed 16 Dec 2017.
19. Ashworth A. Nutrition, food security, and health. In: Kleigman RM, Stanton BF, Schor NF, St Geme III JW, Behrman RE, editors. Nelson textbook of pediatrics. 20th ed. Philadelphia: Elsevier; 2016. p. 295–306.
20. Becher JC, Lasing I. History, examination, basic investigations and procedures. In: Mcintosh N, Helms PJ, Smyth RL, Logan S, editors. Forfar and Arneil's textbook of pediatrics. 7th ed. Edinburgh: Elsevier Limited. p. 115–58.
21. Lissauer T, Macaulay C. History and examination. In: Lissauer T, Carroll W, editors. Illustrated textbook of pediatrics. 5th ed. Edinburgh: Elsevier; 2018. p. 9–26.
22. Turner A, Doraiswamy NV. Paediatric emergencies. In: Goel KM, Gupta DK, editors. Hutchison's pediatrics. 2nd ed. New Delhi: Jaypee Brothers Medical Publishers; 2012. p. 618–38.
23. Reddy VN. Vital signs. In: Greydanus DE, Feinberg AN, Patel DR, Homnick DN, editors. The pediatric diagnostic examination. New York: The McGraw-Hill; 2008. p. 45–58.
24. Thangadorai C. Physical examination. In: Parthasarathy A, Gupta P, Nair M, Menon P, Agarwal RK, Sukumaran T, editors. IAP textbook of pediatrics. 5th ed. New Delhi: Jaypee Brothers Medical Publishers; 2013. p. 7–17.
25. El-Radhi AS, Carroll J. Fever in pediatric practice. Oxford: Blackwell; 1994. p. 68–84.
26. Van der Jagt EW. Fever. In: Adam HM, Foy JM, editors. Signs and symptoms in pediatrics. Elk Grove Village, IL: The American Academy of Pediatrics; 2015. p. 343–59.
27. El-Radhi AS, Carroll J, Klein N, Abbas A. Fever. In: El-Radhi AS, Carroll J, Klein N, editors. Clinical manual of fever in children. New York: Springer; 2009. p. 1–24.
28. Szilagyi PG. Assessing children: infancy through adolescence. In: Bickley LS, Szilagyi PG, editors. Bates' guide to physical examination and history-taking. 11th ed. Philadelphia: Wolters Kluwer Health/Lippincott Williams & Wilkins; 2013. p. 765–891.
29. Potter DE, Hoffman JIE. Systemic hypertension. In: Rudolph AM, Siegel NJ, Rudolph CD, Hostetter MK, Lister G, editors. Rudolph's pediatrics. 21st ed. New York: McGraw-Hill Medical; 2003. p. 1877–86.
30. Dickey BZ, Chiu YE. Evaluation of the patient. In: Kleigman RM, Stanton BF, Schor NF, St Geme III JW, Behrman RE, editors. Nelson textbook of pediatrics. 20th ed. Philadelphia: Elsevier; 2016. p. 3105–13.
31. Zorc JJ, Schwartz MW. Obtaining and presenting a patient history. In: Zorc JJ, Alpern ER, Brown LW, Loomes KM, Marino BS, Mollen CJ, et al., editors. Schwartz's clinical handbook of pediatrics. 5th ed. Philadelphia: Lippincott Williams & Wilkins Business; 2013. p. 1–5.
32. Kinsman SL, Johnston MV. Congenital anomalies of the central nervous system. In: Kleigman RM, Stanton BF, Schor NF, St Geme III JW, Behrman RE, editors. Nelson textbook of pediatrics. 20th ed. Philadelphia: Elsevier; 2016. p. 2802–19.
33. Moses PD, Thomas MM, Koshy B. Diseases of nervous system. In: Goel KM, Gupta DK, editors. Hutchison's pediatrics. 2nd ed. New Delhi: Jaypee Brothers Medical Publishers; 2012. p. 360–98.

34. Goel KM, Carachi R. Pediatric history and examination. In: Goel KM, Gupta DK, editors. Hutchison's pediatrics. 2nd ed. New Delhi: Jaypee Brothers Medical Publishers; 2012. p. 1–17.
35. Magon P. Pearls in clinical pediatrics. New Delhi: Jaypee Brothers Medical Publishers; 2013.
36. Warren AE, Roy DL. Cardiovascular assessment of infants and children. In: Goldbloom RB, editor. Pediatric clinical skills. 4th ed. Philadelphia: Elsevier Saunders; 2011. p. 137–59.
37. Stephenson T, Wallace H, Thomson A. Clinical pediatrics for postgraduate examination. 3rd ed. Elsevier Science: Edinburgh; 2002.
38. Stenson B, Turner S. Babies and children. In: Douglas G, Nicol F, Robertson C, editors. Macleod's clinical examination. 13th ed. Edinburgh: Elsevier; 2013. p. 355–78.
39. Bernstein D. History and physical examination. In: Kleigman RM, Stanton BF, Schor NF, St Geme III JW, Behrman RE, editors. Nelson textbook of pediatrics. 20th ed. Philadelphia: Elsevier; 2016. p. 2163–70.
40. Upton C, Thalange N. Respiration. In: Thalange N, Beach R, Booth D, Jackson L, editors. Pocket essentials of pediatrics. 2nd ed. Edinburgh: Elsevier; 2013. p. 99–117.
41. Weiner DL. Emergency evaluation and immediate management of acute respiratory distress in children. In: Fleisher GR, Wiley JF, editors. UpToDate. 2016. http://www.uptodate.com/contents/emergency-evaluation-and-immediate-management-of-acute-respiratory-distress-in-children. Accessed 9 Feb 2018.
42. Brugha R, Marlais M, Abrahamson E. Pocket tour pediatrics clinical examination. London: JP Medical; 2013.
43. Abend NS. Coma. In: Zorc JJ, Alpern ER, Brown LW, Loomes KM, Marino BS, Mollen CJ, et al., editors. Schwartz's clinical handbook of pediatrics. 5th ed. Philadelphia: Lippincott Williams & Wilkins; 2013. p. 228–240.
44. Khan MA, Pandya A. OSCEs in pediatrics. Edinburgh: Elsevier Science; 2002.
45. Baldwin KD, Wells W, Dormans JP. Clinical evaluation of the child. In: Kleigman RM, Stanton BF, Schor NF, St Geme III JW, Behrman RE, editors. Nelson textbook of pediatrics. 20th ed. Philadelphia: Elsevier; 2016. p. 3242–7.

Appendix

Suggested diagnostic framework

1. **Take a history.**
   - **Identity (patient demographics)**
     - Child's name
     - Age/date of birth
     - Sex
     - Address/ birthplace
     - Nationality, ethnicity/race
     - Name and relationship of the informant
     - Date/time of the interview or admission
     - Source of referral
   - **Chief complaint(s) and duration**
   - **History of present illness**
   - **Past history**
     - Birth history
       Antenatal
       Natal
       Postnatal and neonatal
     - Past medical and surgical history
   - **Medication history**
   - **Developmental history**
     - Gross motor
     - Fine motor and vision
     - Speech, language, and hearing
     - Social, emotional, and behavioral
   - **Immunization history**
   - **Feeding/dietary history**
   - **Family history**
   - **Social history**
   - **Review of systems**

© Springer International Publishing AG, part of Springer Nature 2018
A. Qais Saadoon, *Essential Clinical Skills in Pediatrics*,
https://doi.org/10.1007/978-3-319-92426-7

Suggested diagnostic framework

2. **Summarize the important points in the patient's history.**

3. **Perform a physical examination guided by the patient's history.**
   - **General inspection**
   - **Vital signs**
     Pulse rate, respiratory rate, temperature, blood pressure, and SpO_2
   - **Anthropometric measurements**
     Weight, height or length, head circumference and plot the measurements on an appropriate growth chart
   - **Assessment of hydration status**
   - **Assessment of nutritional status**
   - **Examination of the skin, hair, and nails**
   - **Examination of the head, face, and neck**
   - **Cardiovascular system examination**
     - General physical examination
     - Examination of the precordium
   - **Respiratory system examination**
     - General physical examination
     - Examination of the chest
   - **Gastrointestinal system examination**
     - General physical examination
     - Examination of the abdomen and further examination
   - **Genital examination**
   - **Reticuloendothelial system examination**
   - **Examination of the nervous system**
     - General physical examination
     - Mental status examination
     - Cranial nerves examination
     - Motor system examination
     - Sensory system examination
     - Reflexes and clonus
     - Coordination and cerebellar signs
   - **Musculoskeletal system examination**
     - General physical examination
     - Examination of the joints

4. **Summarize the history and examination findings.**

5. **Generate a differential diagnosis list.**
   - List the most probable diagnoses in the order of their probability.

6. **Perform the relevant investigations, procedures, and consultations.**

7. **Summarize your findings and make a definite diagnosis.**
   - List the important features in the history and physical findings, in addition to the results of the investigations that have been performed on the patient. This may narrow the differential diagnosis list.
   - Modify your list of differential diagnoses accordingly.
   - Make the definite diagnosis.

8. **If uncertain, repeat the above points (1–7) until you reach a definite diagnosis, or consider a provisional diagnosis or watchful waiting.**

9. **Treat the condition.**

10. **Note the patient progress.**
    - Record the investigations that have been done for the patient, the treatment that he/she received, and the current condition (improved, same, deteriorated).

11. **Record the follow-up notes.**

Index

© Springer International Publishing AG, part of Springer Nature 2018
A. Qais Saadoon, *Essential Clinical Skills in Pediatrics*,
https://doi.org/10.1007/978-3-319-92426-7